The

Final Work

ANSWERING HUMANITY'S NEED

Revised and Enlarged 2004

A compilation of inspired counsel
for the preparation of
gospel medical missionaries.

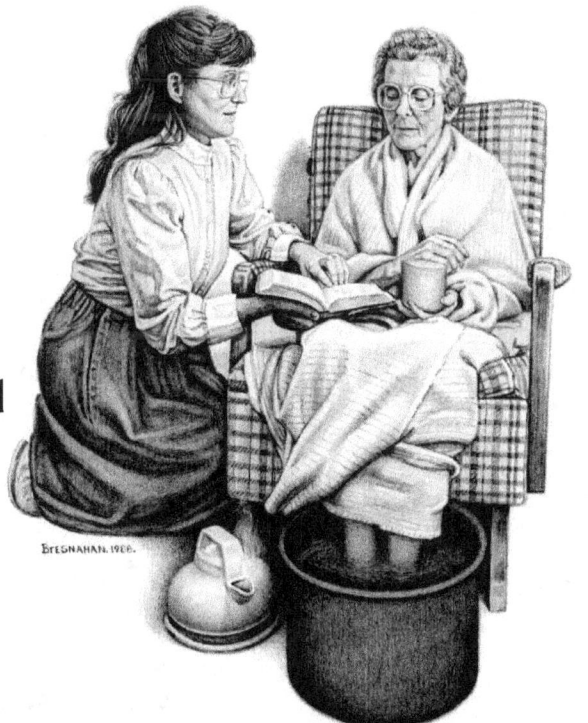

" . . . soon there will be no work done in ministerial lines but medical missionary work."
Counsels on Health, 533.

A great work is to be done in our world,
and human agencies will surely respond to the demand.
And all the requisite talent, courage, perseverance, faith, and tact will
come as they put the armor on.
Mrs. E. G. White.
Bible Echo, September 18, 1899.

Medical missionary work—Christ's end-time work—
is discussed by means of over 500 Spirit of Prophecy quotations.
Excellent for personal and group study
and as a source
for talks and seminars.

Revised and enlarged 1991, 2001, 2004

© 1990, 1991, 2001, 2004
Vernon C. Sparks M.D.

Published
by

DIGITAL INSPIRATION
1481 Reagan Valley Road
Tellico Plains, TN 37385
http://vsdigitalinspiration.com

Contents

Reasons For Reform

My people are destroyed for lack of knowledge. Hosea 4:6.

1. Our first duty toward God and our fellow beings is the establishment and the preservation of our personal physical and mental health.

Counsels on Health, 107–108.

OUR first duty toward God and our fellow beings is that of self-development. Every faculty with which the Creator has endowed us should be cultivated to the highest degree of perfection, that we may be able to do the greatest amount of good of which we are capable. Hence that time is spent to good account which is used in the establishment and preservation of physical and mental health. We cannot afford to dwarf or cripple any function of body or mind. As surely as we do this, we must suffer the consequences.

2. We are to know and to obey the principles that will restore in us the divine image.

The Ministry of Healing, 114–115.

GOD desires us to reach the standard of perfection made possible for us by the gift of Christ. He calls upon us to make our choice on the right side, to connect with heavenly agencies, to adopt principles that will restore in us the divine image. In His written word and in the great book of nature He has revealed the principles of life. It is our work to obtain a knowledge of these principles, and by obedience to cooperate with Him in restoring health to the body as well as to the soul.

3. God is pledged to maintain the health of the human body if we obey His laws and cooperate with Him.

Counsels on Diet and Foods, 17.

THE Creator of man has arranged the living machinery of our bodies. Every function is wonderfully and wisely made. And God pledged Himself to keep this human machinery in healthful action if the human agent will obey His laws and cooperate with God. Every law governing the human machinery is to be considered just as truly divine in origin, in character, and in importance as the word of God. Every careless, inattentive action, any abuse put upon the Lord's wonderful mechanism by disregarding His specified laws in the human habitation, is a violation of God's law. We may behold and admire the work of God in the natural world, but the human habitation, is the most wonderful.

4. If we disobey the natural laws of our being, we will tend to break the ten commandments.

Christian Temperance and Bible Hygiene, 53.

IT IS truly a sin to violate the laws of our being as it is to break the ten commandments. To do either is to break God's laws. Those who transgress the law of God in their physical organism, will be inclined to violate the law of God spoken from Sinai.

5. The truly converted will, through obedience to natural law, seek to avoid physical, mental, and moral feebleness.

Testimonies, vol. 6, 369–370.

WHEN men and women are truly converted, they will conscientiously regard the laws of life that God has established in their being, thus seeking to avoid physical, mental, and moral feebleness. Obedience to these laws must be made a matter of personal duty. We ourselves must suffer the ills of violated law. We must answer to God for our habits and practices. Therefore, the question for us is not, "What will the world say?" but, "How shall I, claiming to be a Christian, treat the habitation God has given me? Shall I work for my highest temporal and spiritual good by keeping my body as a temple for the indwelling of the Holy Spirit, or shall I sacrifice myself to the world's ideas and practices?"

6. Ignorance of natural law is the major cause of disease.

Counsels on Diet and Foods, 19.

THE majority of diseases which the human family have been and still are suffering under, they have created by ignorance of their own organic laws.

7. We are to give our body as a healthy, living sacrifice to God for a temple of the Holy Ghost.

Counsels on Health, 121.

GOD requires the body to be rendered a living sacrifice to Him, not a dead or a dying sacrifice. The offerings of the ancient Hebrews were to be without blemish, and will it be pleasing to God to accept a human offering that is filled with disease and corruption? He tells us that our body is the temple of the Holy Ghost; and He requires us to take care of this temple, that it may be a fit habitation for His Spirit. The apostle Paul gives us this admonition: "Ye are not your own; for ye are bought with a price; therefore, glorify God in your body and in your spirit, which are God's." All should be very careful to preserve the body in the best condition of health, that they may render to God perfect service, and do their duty in the family and in society.

8. We rob our families and neighbors, as well as God, when we disobey the laws of health.

Testimonies, vol. 3, 164–165.

OUR first duty, one which we owe to God, to ourselves, and to our fellow men, is to obey the laws of God, which include the laws of health. If we are sick, we impose a weary tax upon our friends, and unfit ourselves for discharging our duties to our families and to our neighbors. And when premature death is the result of our violation of nature's law, we bring sorrow and suffering to others; we deprive our neighbors of the help we ought to render them in living; we rob our families of the comfort and help we might render them, and rob God of the service He claims of us to advance His glory. Then, are we not, in the worst sense, transgressors of God's law?

9. It is impossible to indulge appetite and also to attain to Christian perfection.

Testimonies, vol. 2, 399–400.

ALL who are partakers of the divine nature will escape the corruption that is in the world through lust. It is impossible for those who indulge the appetite to attain to Christian perfection.

10. Heaven has sent us the light of health reform in order that we might be sanctified through the truth.

Counsels on Health, 120–121.

OUR heavenly Father sent the light of health reform to guard against the evils resulting from a debased appetite, that those who love purity and holiness may know how to use with discretion the good things He has provided for them, and that by exercising temperance in daily life, they may be sanctified through the truth.

11. Health reform will draw a distinct line between those who serve God and those who serve themselves.

Testimonies, vol. 9, 158.

LET those who are teachers and leaders in our cause take their stand firmly on Bible ground in regard to health reform and give a straight testimony to those who believe we are living in the last days of this earth's history. A line of distinction must be drawn between those who serve God, and those who serve themselves.

12. It requires stern work to secure the best physical health, in order to have the mental clearness to discern between good and evil.

Christian Temperance and Bible Hygiene, 25.

THERE is work for us to do—stern, earnest work. All our habits, tastes, and inclinations must be educated in harmony with the laws of life and health. By this means we may secure the very best physical conditions, and have mental clearness to discern between the evil and the good.

13. To set aside a "Thus saith the Lord" is to lead others astray, and its seriousness will be revealed in the judgment.

Review and Herald, vol. 1, 253.

THERE are many among professed Christians today who would decide that Daniel was too particular, and would pronounce him narrow and bigoted. They consider the matter of eating and drinking of too little consequence to require such a decided stand, one involving the probable sacrifice of every earthly advantage. But those who reason thus will find in the day of judgment that they turned from God's express requirements, and set up their own opinion as a standard of right and wrong. They will find that what seemed to them unimportant was not so regarded of God. His requirements should be sacredly obeyed. Those who accept and obey one of His precepts because it is convenient to do so, while they reject another because its observance would require a sacrifice, lower the standard of right, and by their example lead others to lightly regard the holy law of God. "Thus saith the Lord" is to be our rule in all things.

14. Strict compliance to the laws of health, as well as wisdom and strength from God, are essential to the reaching of the highest standard in moral and intellectual attainments.

Review and Herald, vol. 1, 253.

HERE is a lesson for all, but especially for the young. A strict compliance with the requirements of God is beneficial to the health of body and mind. In order to reach the highest standard of moral and intellectual attainments, it is necessary to seek wisdom and strength from God, and to observe strict temperance in all the habits of life.

15. The latter rain will be poured out only upon those who have had prior victory over wrong health habits.

Testimonies, vol. 1, 619.

I WAS shown that if God's people make no efforts on their part, but wait for the refreshing to come upon them and remove their wrongs and correct their errors; if they depend upon that to cleanse themselves from all filthiness of the flesh and spirit, and fit them to engage in the loud cry of the third angel, they will be found wanting. The refreshing or power of God comes only on those who have prepared themselves for it by doing the work which God bids them, namely, cleansing themselves from all filthiness of the flesh and spirit, perfecting holiness in the fear of God.

16. There will be a wonderful change in religious experience when the continual backsliding in health reform ceases.

Counsels on Health, 578–579.

THE failure to follow sound principles has marred the history of God's people. There has been a continual backsliding in health reform and as a result God is dishonored by a great lack of spirituality.

Far better give up the name of Christian than make a profession and at the same time indulge appetites which strengthen unholy passion. . . . When they break away from all health-destroying indulgences they will have a clearer perception of what constitutes true godliness. A wonderful change will be seen in the religious experience.

17. A restricted diet without a transformed appetite is not true temperance.

Special Testimonies, Series A, 54.

NO MERE restriction of your diet will cure your diseased appetite. Brother and Sister _____ will not practice temperance in all things until their hearts are transformed by the grace of God.

18. Only true health reformers will meet the mind of God.

Counsels on Diet and Foods, 36.

IF WE move from principle in these things, if we observe strict rules of diet, if as Christians we educate our tastes after God's plan, we shall exert an influence which will meet the mind of God. The question is, "Are we willing to be true health reformers?"

19. True health reform will have to be done before we can stand before God a perfected people.

Testimonies, vol. 9, 153–154.

THOSE who have received instruction regarding the evils of the use of flesh foods, tea and coffee, and rich and unhealthful food preparations, and who are determined to make a covenant with God by sacrifice, will not continue to indulge their appetite for food that they know to be unhealthful. God demands that the appetites be cleansed, and that self-denial be practiced in regard to those things which are not good. This is a work that will have to be done before His people can stand before Him a perfected people.

20. Health reform, rather than a stumbling block, is a stepping-stone to heaven.

Testimonies, vol. 1, 546.

SAID the angel, "Abstain from fleshly lusts which war against the soul." You have stumbled at the health reform. It appears to you to be a needless appendix to the truth. It is not so; it is a part of the truth. Here is a work before you which will come closer and be more trying than anything which has yet been brought to bear upon you. While you hesitate and stand back, failing to lay hold upon the blessing which it is your privilege to receive, you suffer loss. You are stumbling over the very blessing which heaven has placed in your path to make progress less difficult. Satan presents this before you in the most objectionable light, that you may combat that which would prove the greatest benefit to you, which would be for your physical and spiritual health.

21. God calls us to repent and to cease from dwarfing our physical, mental, and spiritual powers.

Evangelism, 262.

MANY have done the body much injury by a disregard of the laws of life, and they may never recover from the effects of their neglect; but even now they may repent and be converted. Man has tried to be wiser than God. He has become a law unto himself. God calls upon us to give attention to His requirements, no longer to dishonor Him by dwarfing the physical, mental, and spiritual capabilities.

22. All improvements here of our mental powers are taken with us to heaven.

Manuscript Releases, vol. 9, 21.

ETERNITY is before us. All improvements we make here of our mental powers, all the high attainments we make in refining and elevating ourselves by connecting closely with heaven, will be translated with us, while if we dwarf our capabilities by inaction, if we deteriorate our talents, which are susceptible of the highest cultivation, we cannot in the better world redeem that past neglect of self-culture, that great loss.

Some may be saved as by fire. Their useless life has brought to them infinite loss. We should make improvement in this life, all that we can by the help and grace of God, knowing we can take these improvements with us into heaven.

Manuscript Releases, vol. 3, 353.

REASONING we must have. It is one of the great masterly talents entrusted to the human agent, and is a great advantage at every step we advance from earth to heaven. The faculty of reasoning, trained and cultivated as a precious, entrusted gift, will be taken to heaven with all its improvements and sanctified abilities, to be perfected more and more in the heavenly school above.

23. The more fully we surrender spirit, soul, mind, and body to the Holy Spirit, the more fragrant will be our offering to Him.

The Seventh-day Adventist Bible Commentary, vol. 7, 909.

GOD would have us realize that He has a right to mind, soul, body, and spirit to all that we possess. We are His by creation and by redemption. As our Creator, He claims our entire service. As our Redeemer, He has a claim of love as well as of right—of love without a parallel. . . . Our bodies, our souls, our lives, are His, not only because they are His free gift, but because He constantly supplies us with His benefits, and gives us strength to use our faculties. . . .

Those who are sons of God will represent Christ in character. Their works will be perfumed by the infinite tenderness, compassion, love and purity of the Son of God. And the more completely mind and body are yielded to the Holy Spirit, the greater will be the fragrance of our offering to Him.

Diet and Spirituality

If any man will do his will, he shall know of the doctrine. John 7:17.

24. There is a close sympathy between physical health and spirituality.

Counsels on Health, 67.

LET none who profess godliness regard with indifference the health of the body, and flatter themselves that intemperance is no sin, and will not affect their spirituality. A close sympathy exists between the physical and the moral nature.

25. Indulgence of appetite makes sanctification of the body and spirit impossible.

The Health Reformer, 181.

IT IS not possible for us to glorify God while living in violation of the laws of life. The heart cannot possibly maintain consecration to God while lustful appetite is indulged. A diseased body and disordered intellect, because of continual indulgence in hurtful lust, make sanctification of the body and spirit impossible.

26. It is a sacred duty to love the Lord more than our appetites.

Testimonies, vol. 2, 70.

IT IS a duty to know how to preserve the body in the very best condition of health, and it is a sacred duty to live up to the light which God has graciously given. If we close our eyes to the light for fear we shall see our wrongs, which we are unwilling to forsake, our sins are not lessened, but increased. If light is turned from in one case, it will be disregarded in another. It is just as much sin to violate the laws of our being as to break one of the ten commandments, for we cannot do either without breaking God's law. We cannot love the Lord with all our heart, mind, soul, and strength while we are loving our appetites, our tastes, a great deal better than we love the Lord.

27. Indulged appetite is the greatest hindrance to sanctification.

Testimonies, vol. 9, 156.

WE NEED to learn that indulged appetite is the greatest hindrance to mental improvement and soul sanctification.

28. Many lose more sacred Sabbath blessings than they realize because of their overeating.

The Ministry of Healing, 307.

WE SHOULD not provide for the Sabbath a more liberal supply or a greater variety of food than for other days. Instead of this, the food should be more simple, and less should be eaten, in order that the mind may be clear and vigorous to comprehend spiritual things. A clogged stomach means a clogged brain. The most precious words may be heard and not appreciated, because the mind is confused by an improper diet. By overeating on the Sabbath, many do more than they think, to unfit themselves for receiving the benefit of its sacred opportunities.

29. Overeating at camp meetings often creates lethargy in the appreciation of eternal matters.

Testimonies, vol. 5, 162–164.

I HAVE been shown that some of our camp meetings are far from being what the Lord designed they should be. . . . Often the stomach is overburdened with food which is seldom as plain and simple as that eaten at home, where the amount of exercise taken is double or treble. This causes the mind to be in such a lethargy that it is difficult to appreciate eternal things, and the meeting closes, and they are disappointed in not having enjoyed more of the Spirit of God.

30. Indulgence in wrong eating habits will lead to unfitness for the finishing touch of immortality.

Testimonies, vol. 2, 66.

YOU need clear, energetic minds, in order to appreciate the exalted character of the truth, to value the atonement, and to place the right estimate upon eternal things. If you pursue a wrong course, and indulge in wrong habits of eating, and thereby weaken the intellectual powers, you will not place that high estimate upon salvation and eternal life which will inspire you to conform your life to the life of Christ; you will not make those earnest, self-sacrificing efforts for entire conformity to the will of God, which His word requires and which are necessary to give you a moral fitness for the finishing touch of immortality.

31. A weakening of our physical powers decreases our spiritual eyesight and our will power.

Christ's Object Lessons, 346.

ANYTHING that lessens physical strength enfeebles the mind, and makes it less capable of discriminating between right and wrong. We become less capable of choosing the good, and have less strength of will to do that which we know to be right.

The misuse of our physical powers shortens the period of time in which our lives can be used for the glory of God. And it unfits us to accomplish the work God has given us to do.

32. Christ will not reach low enough to raise those who persist in self-gratification.

Spiritual Gifts, vol. 4, 148–149.

THOSE who bring disease upon themselves, by self-gratification, have not healthy bodies and minds. They cannot weigh the evidences of truth, and comprehend the requirements of God. Our Saviour will not reach His arm low enough to raise such from their degraded state, while they persist in pursuing a course to sink themselves still lower.

33. Imprudent eating leads to wrong decisions regarding the Lord's work.

Counsels on Diet and Foods, 53.

WHAT a pity it is that often, when the greatest self-denial should be exercised, the stomach is crowded with a mass of unhealthful food, which lies there to decompose. The affliction of the stomach affects the brain. The imprudent eater does not realize that he is disqualifying himself for giving wise counsel, disqualifying himself for laying plans for the best advancement of the work of God. But this is so. He cannot discern spiritual things, and in council meetings, when he should say Yea and Amen, he says Nay. He makes propositions that are wide of the mark. The food he has eaten has benumbed his brain power.

34. Eden was lost due to indulged appetite, and its restoration must begin with the reformation of man's physical habits.

Testimonies, vol. 3, 486–487.

CHRIST knew that in order to successfully carry forward the plan of salvation He must commence the work of redeeming man just where the ruin began. Adam fell by the indulgence of appetite. In order to impress upon man his obligations to obey the law of God, Christ began His work of redemption by reforming the physical habits of man. The declension in virtue and the degeneracy of the race are chiefly attributable to the indulgence of perverted appetite.

35. Ministers especially must guard their eating habits in order to enjoy the Holy Spirit's blessings upon their spiritual labors.

Counsels on Diet and Foods, 55–56.

MINISTERS, above all others, should economize the strength of brain and nerve. They should avoid all food or drink that has a tendency to irritate or excite the nerves. Excitement will be followed by depression; overindulgence will cloud the mind, and render thought difficult and confused. No man can become a successful workman in spiritual things until he observes strict temperance in his dietetic habits. God cannot let His Holy Spirit rest upon those who, while they know how they should eat for health, persist in a course that will enfeeble mind and body.

36. Health habits have a direct bearing upon our spiritual growth.

The Youth's Instructor, 172.

EATING, drinking, and dressing all have a direct bearing upon our spiritual advancement.

37. Moral health is affected by our habits of eating, drinking, and dressing.

Review and Herald, vol. 1, 254.

THIS is true sanctification. It is not merely a theory, an emotion, or a form of words, but a living, active principle, entering into the everyday life. It requires that our habits of eating, drinking, and dressing be such as to secure the preservation of physical, mental, and moral health, that we may present to the Lord our bodies, not an offering corrupted by wrong habits, but "a living sacrifice, holy, acceptable unto God.".

38. Those who value Christ's sacrifice will choose firm denial of appetite and passion.

Testimonies, vol. 3, 491.

AS OUR first parents lost Eden through the indulgence of appetite, our only hope of regaining Eden is through the firm denial of appetite and passion. Abstemiousness in diet, and control of all the passions, will preserve the intellect and give mental and moral vigor, enabling men to bring all their propensities under the control of the higher powers, and to discern between right and wrong, the sacred and the common. All who have a true sense of the sacrifice made by Christ in leaving His home in heaven to come to this world that He might by His own life show man how to resist temptation, will cheerfully deny itself and choose to be partakers with Christ of His sufferings.

39. Indulgence in appetite will cause many of us to fall in the time of trouble.

Review and Herald, October 21, 1884.

THE reason why many of us will fall in the time of trouble is because of laxity in temperance and indulgence of appetite.

Moses preached a great deal on this subject, and the reason the people did not go through to the promised land was because of repeated indulgence of appetite. Nine-tenths of the wickedness among the children of today is caused by intemperance in eating and drinking. Adam and Eve lost Eden through the indulgence of appetite, and we can only regain it by the denial of the same.

40. The failure to control appetite and passions will result in believing that Satan's snares are providences of God.

Testimonies, vol. 3, 491.

THE fear of the Lord is the beginning of wisdom. Those who overcome as Christ overcame will need to constantly guard themselves against the temptations of Satan. The appetite and passions should be restricted and under the control of enlightened conscience, that the intellect may be unimpaired, the perceptive powers clear, so that the workings of Satan and his snares may not be interpreted to be the providence of God. Many desire the final reward and victory which are to be given to overcomers, but are not willing to endure toil, privation, and denial of self, as did their Redeemer. It is only through obedience and continual effort that we shall overcome as Christ overcame.

41. Victory over appetite is the key to victory over Satan.

Testimonies, vol. 3, 491–492.

THE controlling power of appetite will prove the ruin of thousands, when, if they had conquered on this point, they would have had moral power to gain the victory over every other temptation of Satan. But those who are slaves to appetite will fail in perfecting Christian character. The continual transgression of man for six thousand years has brought sickness, pain, and death as its fruits. And as we near the close of time, Satan's temptation to indulge appetite will be more powerful and more difficult to overcome.

42. Errors in eating and drinking lead to errors in thoughts and actions.

Review and Herald, vol. 1, 254.

ANY habit which does not promote healthful action in the human system, degrades the higher and nobler faculties. Wrong habits of eating and drinking lead to errors in thought and action. Indulgence of appetite strengthens the animal propensities, giving them the ascendance over the mental and spiritual powers.

43. We must choose those foods which best nourish our physical, intellectual, and moral health.

Testimonies, vol. 2, 352.

IF EVER there was a time when the diet should be of the most simple kind, it is now. Meat should not be placed before our children. Its influence is to excite and strengthen the lower passions, and has a tendency to deaden the moral powers. Grains and fruits prepared free from grease, and in as natural a condition as possible, should be the food for the tables of all who claim to be preparing for translation to heaven. The less feverish the diet, the more easily can the passions be controlled. Gratification of taste should not be consulted irrespective of physical, intellectual, or moral health.

44. Victorious warfare over appetite and passions

and thus over Satan is open to all who will engage in it.

Testimonies, vol. 4, 35–36.

THERE is no encouragement given to any of the sons or daughters of Adam that they may become victorious overcomers in the Christian warfare unless they decide to practice temperance in all things. If they do this, they will not fight as one that beateth the air.

If Christians will keep the body in subjection, and bring all their appetites and passions under the control of enlightened conscience, feeling it a duty that they owe to God and to their neighbors to obey the laws which govern health and life, they will have the blessing of physical and mental vigor. They will have moral power to engage in the warfare against Satan; and in the name of Him who conquered appetite in their behalf, they may be more than conquerors on their own account. This warfare is open to all who will engage in it.

45. Total obedience is the only true sign of sanctification.

The Seventh-day Adventist Bible Commentary, vol. 7, 908.

OBEDIENCE to all the commandments of God is the only true sign of sanctification. Disobedience is the sign of disloyalty and apostasy.

46. Unhealthful practices must be overcome in order for man to be sanctified.

The Seventh-day Adventist Bible Commentary, vol. 7, 909.

THE truth must sanctify the whole man his mind, his thoughts, his heart, his strength. His vital powers will not be consumed upon his own lustful practices. These must be overcome, or they will overcome him.

Health Reform and the Third Angel's Message

Know ye not that ye are the temple of God. 1Corinthians 3:16.

47. Health reform is the hand of the third angel's message.

Testimonies, vol. 3, 161–162.

DECEMBER 10, 1871, I was shown that the health reform is one branch of the great work which is to fit a people for the coming of the Lord, It is as closely connected with the third angel's message as the hand is with the body.

48. The explanation of and the exhortation to obey the laws of nature are a part of the final message to fallen man.

Testimonies, vol. 3, 161.

TO MAKE plain natural law, and urge the obedience of it, is the work that accompanies the third angel's message, to prepare a people for the coming of the Lord.

49. The public mind is to be deeply stirred regarding health reform in order to enable them to discern spiritual truth.

Testimonies, vol. 3, 162.

HE [God] designs that the great subject of health reform shall be agitated, and the public mind deeply stirred to investigate; for it is impossible for men and women, with all their sinful, health-destroying, brain enervating habits, to discern sacred truth, through which they are to be sanctified, refined, elevated, and made fit for the society of heavenly angels in the kingdom of glory.

50. Health reform is one of the great branches of work to prepare for Christ's coming.

Testimonies, vol. 3, 61.

FOR years the Lord has been calling the attention of His people to health reform. This is one of the great branches of the work of preparation for the coming of the Son of man.

51. The full third angel's message has an all-pervasive role for health reform, but a nondomineering role for health work.

Testimonies, vol. 6, 327.

WHEN the third angel's message is received in its fullness, health reform will be given its place in the councils of the conference, in the work of the church, in the home, at the table, and in all the household arrangements. Then the right arm will serve and protect the body.

But while the health work has its place in the promulgation of the third angel's message, its advocates must not in any way strive to make it take the place of the message.

52. By example and by word the ministry are to present health reform to all converts as an integral part of the third angel's message.

Testimonies, vol. 1, 469–470.

ONE important part of the work of the ministry is to faithfully present to the people the health reform, as it stands connected with the third angel's message, as a part and parcel of the same work. They should not fail to adopt it themselves, and should urge it upon all who profess to believe the truth.

53. We each have a personal, individual work of health reform, essential in preparation for the loud cry of the third angel.

Testimonies, vol. 1, 486.

THE health reform, I was shown, is a part of the third angel's message, and is just as closely connected with it as are the arm and hand with the human body. I saw that we as a people must make an advance move in this great work. Ministers and people must act in concert. God's people are not prepared for the loud cry of the third angel. They have a work to do for themselves which they should not leave for God to do for them. He has left this work for them to do. It is an individual work; one cannot do it for another.

54. Health principles are in no way to be independent of or to take the place of God's final message.

Counsels on Diet and Foods, 75.

THE proclamation of the third angel's message, the commandments of God and the testimony of Jesus, is the burden of our work. The message is to be proclaimed with a loud cry, and is to go to the whole world. The presentation of health principles must be united with this message, but must not in any case be independent of it, or in any way take the place of it.

55. Health reform is to have a prominent, restoring influence in God's final message.

Counsels on Diet and Foods, 75.

HEALTH reform is to stand out more prominently in the proclamation of the third angel's message. The principles of health reform are found in the Word of God. The gospel of health is to be firmly linked with the ministry of the Word. It is the Lord's design that the restoring influence of health reform shall be a part of the last great effort to proclaim the gospel message.

56. We would have a far greater influence than we do if we would practice and preach health reform with a greater interest.

Christian Temperance and Bible Hygiene, 121–122.

IF THE church would manifest a greater interest in the reforms through which God Himself is seeking to fit them for His coming, their influence would be far greater than it now is. God has spoken to His people, and He designs that they shall hear and obey His voice. Although the health reform is not the third angel's message, it is closely connected with it. Those who proclaim the message should teach health reform also. It is a subject that we must understand, in order to be prepared for the events that are close upon us, and it should have a prominent place.

57. God's purpose for health reform is to relieve human suffering, as well as to purify His people.

Testimonies, vol. 9, 112–113.

THE work of health reform is the Lord's means for lessening suffering in our world and for purifying His church.

58. True sanctification involves a sincere regard for all of God's commandments.

Review and Herald, vol. 2, 80.

TRUE sanctification will be evidenced by a conscientious regard for all the commandments of God, by a careful, improvement of every talent, by a circumspect conversation, by revealing in every act the meekness of Christ.

59. True Christian experience brings soul and body into harmony with God as a fit temple for the Holy Spirit.

The Seventh-day Adventist Bible Commentary, vol. 7, 909.

SANCTIFICATION how many understand its full meaning? The mind is befogged by sensual malaria. . . . What might not men and women have been had they realized that the treatment of the body has everything to do with the vigor and purity of mind and heart.

The true Christian obtains an experience which brings holiness. He is without a spot of guilt upon the conscience, or a taint of corruption upon the soul. . . . The will of God has become his will, pure, elevated, refined, and sanctified. His countenance reveals the light of heaven. His body is a fit temple for the Holy Spirit. Holiness adorns his character. God can commune with him; for soul and body are in harmony with God.

The True Remedies

The true remedies—the eight natural remedies—are the divine principles of healthful living which will govern the well-being of the redeemed throughout all ages. Their present-day adoption affords now a foretaste of that future life.

60. *Ministry of Healing*, 127.
PURE AIR, SUNLIGHT, ABSTEMIOUSNESS, REST, EXERCISE, PROPER DIET, the use of WATER, TRUST IN DIVINE POWER—these are THE TRUE REMEDIES. Every person should have a knowledge of nature's remedial agencies and how to apply them. [All emphasis supplied unless otherwise noted].

61. *Medical Ministry*, 230.
I SHOULD do a very unwise thing to enter a cool room when in a perspiration; I should show myself an unwise steward to allow myself to sit in a draft and thus expose myself so as to take cold. I should be unwise to sit with cold feet and limbs and thus drive back the blood from the extremities to the brain or internal organs. I should always protect my feet in damp weather. I should eat regularly of the most healthful food which will make the best quality of blood, and I should not work intemperately if it is in my power to avoid doing so. And when I violate the laws God has established in my being, I am to repent and reform, and place myself in the most favorable condition under the doctors God has provided—PURE AIR, pure WATER, and the healing, precious SUNLIGHT.

62. *Medical Ministry*, 225.
THE sick should be educated to have confidence in nature's great blessings which God has provided; and the most effective remedies for disease are pure soft WATER, the blessed God-given SUNSHINE coming into the rooms of the invalids, living outdoors as much as possible, having healthful EXERCISE, eating and drinking FOODS that are prepared in the most healthful manner.

63. *Counsels on Health*, 166.
LIFE in the open air is good for body and mind. It is God's medicine for the restoration of health. PURE AIR, good WATER, SUNSHINE, the beautiful surroundings of nature—these are His means for restoring the sick to health in natural ways. To the sick it is worth more than silver or gold to lie in the sunshine or in the shade of the trees.

The True Remedies—I
Pure Air

64. Air stimulates the whole body, strengthening it to resist disease.

Testimonies, vol. 1, 701.

AIR is the free blessing of Heaven, calculated to electrify the whole system. Without it the system will be filled with disease and become dormant, languid, feeble.

65. Pure, fresh air has a beneficial effect upon the nerves, the blood, the mind, the appetite, the digestion, and upon the sleep.

Testimonies, vol. 1, 702.

AIR, air, the precious boon of heaven which all may have, will bless you with its invigorating influence if you will not refuse it entrance. Welcome it, cultivate a love for it, and it will prove a precious soother of the nerves. Air must be in constant circulation to be kept pure. The influence of pure, fresh air is to cause the blood to circulate healthfully through the system. It refreshes the body and tends to render it strong and healthy, while at the same time its influence is decidedly felt upon the mind, imparting a degree of composure and serenity. It excites the appetite, and renders the digestion of food more perfect, and induces sound and sweet sleep.

66. Good blood—cleansed and vitalized by pure air—is essential to good health.

The Ministry of Healing, 271.

IN ORDER to have good health, we must have good blood; for the blood is the current of life. It repairs waste, and nourishes the body. When supplied with the proper food elements and when cleansed and vitalized by contact with pure air, it carries life and vigor to every part of the system. The more perfect the circulation, the better will this work be accomplished.

67. Good blood is dependent upon full, deep inspirations of pure air.

The Ministry of Healing, 272.

IN ORDER to have good blood, we must breathe well. Full, deep inspirations of pure air, which fill the lungs with oxygen, purify the blood. They impart to it a bright color and send it, a life-giving current, to every part of the body. A good respiration soothes the nerves; it stimulates the appetite, and renders digestion more perfect; and it induces sound, refreshing sleep.

68. Correct posture is essential to proper breathing and is to be insisted upon.

Education, 198.

AMONG the first things to be aimed at should be a correct position, both in sitting and in standing. God made man upright, and He desires him to possess not only the physical but the mental and moral benefit, the grace and dignity and self-possession, the courage and self-reliance, which an erect bearing so greatly tends to promote. Let the teacher give instruction on this point by example and by precept. Show what a correct position is, and insist that it shall be maintained.

69. Proper breathing and the correct use of the voice are next in importance to good posture in the proper use of the respiratory organs.

Education, 198.

NEXT in importance to right position are respiration and vocal culture. The one who sits and stands erect is more likely than others to breathe properly. But the teacher should impress upon his pupils the importance of deep breathing. Show how the healthy action of the respiratory organs, assisting the circulation of the blood, invigorates the whole system, excites the appetite, promotes digestion, and induces sound, sweet sleep, thus not only refreshing the body, but soothing and tranquilizing the mind. And while the importance of deep breathing is shown, the practice should be insisted upon. Let exercises be given which will promote this, and see that the habit becomes established.

70. The use of the abdominal muscles is essential in proper breathing and in the proper use of the voice.

Education, 199.

THE training of the voice has an important place in physical culture, since it tends to expand and strengthen the lungs, and thus to ward off disease. To insure correct delivery in reading and speaking, see that the abdominal muscles have full play in breathing, and that the respiratory organs are unrestricted. Let the strain come on the muscles of the abdomen, rather than on those of throat. Great weariness and serious disease of the throat and lungs may thus be prevented. Careful attention should be given to securing distinct articulation, smooth, well-modulated tones, and a not-too rapid delivery. This will not only promote health, but will add greatly to the agreeableness and efficiency of the student's work.

71. Tight clothing interferes with breathing, digestion, and circulation, and thus lessens the physical and mental powers.

Education, 199.

IN TEACHING these things a golden opportunity is afforded for showing the folly and wickedness of tight-lacing, and every other practice that restricts vital action. An almost endless train of disease results from unhealthful modes of dress, and careful instruction of this point should be given. Impress upon the pupils the danger of allowing the clothing to weigh on the hips or to compress any organ of the body. The dress should be so arranged that a full respiration can be taken, and the arms be raised above the head without difficulty. The cramping of the lungs not only prevents their development, but hinders the processes of digestion and circulation, and thus weakens the whole body. All such practices lessen both physical and mental power, thus hindering the student's advancement, and often preventing his success.

72. Stooping and tight clothing results in habitual shallow breathing, which is the underlying cause of many health problems.

The Ministry of Healing, 272–273.

THE lungs should be allowed the greatest freedom possible. Their capacity is developed by free action; it diminishes if they are cramped and compressed. Hence the ill effects of the practice so common, especially in sedentary pursuits, of stooping at one's work. In this position it is impossible to breathe deeply. Superficial breathing soon becomes a habit, and the lungs lose their power to expand. A similar effect is produced by tight lacing. Sufficient room is not given to the lower part of the chest; the abdominal muscles, which were designed to aid in breathing, do not have full play, and the lungs are restricted in their action.

Thus an insufficient supply of oxygen is received. The blood moves sluggishly. The waste, poisonous matter, which should be thrown off in the exhalations from the lungs, is retained, and the blood becomes impure. Not only the lungs, but the stomach, liver, and brain are affected. The skin becomes sallow, digestion is retarded; the heart is depressed; the brain is clouded; the thoughts are confused; gloom settles upon the spirits; the whole system becomes depressed and inactive, and peculiarly susceptible to disease.

73. Clothing should obstruct neither the circulation nor the respiration.

The Ministry of Healing, 293.

EVERY article of dress should fit easily, obstructing neither the circulation of the blood nor a free, full, natural respiration. Everything worn should be so loose that when the arms are raised the clothing will be correspondingly lifted.

74. The clothing should be suspended from the shoulders and roomy enough that it can be gotten on and off without tugging and pulling.

Child Guidance, 426.

TIGHT bands or waists hinder the action of the heart and lungs and should be avoided. No part of the body should at any time be made uncomfortable by clothing that compresses any organ or restricts its freedom of movement. The clothing of all children should be loose enough to admit of the freest and fullest respiration, and so arranged that the shoulders will support its weight.

Daughters of God, 175–176.

IT IS my positive orders that sleeves and waist be made loose and not so tight that there will be compression anywhere. Every muscle must be left free to do its work without having to strain the cloth to use the arms freely. . . .

Give the lungs ample room to exercise, the heart ample room to do its work without one particle of pinching. . . . I am decided that these close, skin-tight sleeves cannot be wise or healthful, and whether it be fashionable or unfashionable, I advise that they not be made after the tight order. Read this to the ones who do my sewing. . . .

I give positive orders that it shall be made roomy and not so tight that she cannot get it on or off without tugging and pulling.

75. Poorly ventilated rooms are another cause of the many illnesses resulting from improper respiration.

Testimonies, vol. 1, 702–703.

THE effects produced by living in close, ill-ventilated rooms are these: The system becomes weak and unhealthy, the circulation is depressed, the blood moves sluggishly through the system because it is not purified and vitalized by the pure, invigorating air of heaven. The mind becomes depressed and gloomy, while the whole system is enervated; and fevers and other acute diseases are liable to be generated. Your careful exclusion of external air and fear of free ventilation leave you to breathe the corrupt, unwholesome air which is exhaled from the lungs of those staying in these rooms, and which is poisonous, unfit for the support of life. The body becomes relaxed, the skin becomes sallow, digestion is retarded, and the system is peculiarly sensitive to the influence of cold. A slight exposure produces serious diseases. Great care should be exercised not to sit in a draft or in a cold room when weary, or when in a perspiration. You should so accustom yourself to the air that you will not be under the necessity of having the mercury higher than sixty-five degrees.

76. The polluted air of the cities is very unhealthful.

Testimonies, vol. 7, 81–82.

THE very atmosphere of the cities is polluted. . . . From the standpoint of health the smoke and dust of the cities are very objectionable.

77. The cities with their impure air and generally unhealthy environment are especially undesirable for the sick.

The Ministry of Healing, 262–263.

THE noise and excitement and confusion of the cities, their constrained and artificial life, are most wearisome and exhausting to the sick. The air, laden with smoke and dust, with poisonous gases, and with germs of disease, is a peril to life. The sick, for the most part shut within four walls, come almost to feel as if they were prisoners in their rooms. They look out on houses and pavements and hurrying crowds, with perhaps not even a glimpse of blue sky or sunshine, or grass or flower or tree. Shut up in this way, they brood over their suffering and sorrow, and become a prey to their own sad thoughts.

78. Foul air is only one of the many perils to health in the cities.

The Ministry of Healing, 365.

THE physical surroundings in the cities are often a peril to health. The constant liability to contact with disease, the prevalence of foul air, impure water, impure food, the crowded, dark, unhealthful dwellings, are some of the many evils to be met.

79. Home sites need a free circulation of air that is purified by the sunlight and free from the contamination of decaying vegetation.

Counsels on Health, 58.

SHADE trees and shrubbery too close and dense around a house are unhealthful; for they prevent a free circulation of air, and shut out the rays of the sun. In consequence of this, dampness gathers in the house. Especially in wet seasons the sleeping rooms become damp, and those who occupy them are troubled with rheumatism, neuralgia, and lung complaints which generally end in consumption. Numerous shade trees cast off many leaves, which, if not immediately removed, decay, and poison the atmosphere. A yard beautified with trees and shrubbery, at a proper distance from the house, has a happy, cheerful influence upon the family, and, if well taken care of, will prove no injury to health. Dwellings, if possible, should be built upon high and dry ground. If a house is built where water settles around it, remaining for a time, and then drying away, a poisonous miasma arises, and fever and ague, sore throat, lung diseases, and fevers will be the result.

80. Poor health can be the result of poorly drained home sites.

The Ministry of Healing, 274.

SO FAR as possible, all buildings intended for human habitation should be placed on high, well-drained ground. This will insure a dry site, and prevent the danger of disease from dampness and miasma. This matter is often too lightly regarded. Continuous ill-health, serious diseases, and many deaths result from the dampness and malaria of low-lying, ill-drained situations.

81. No unclean or decaying matter should be allowed around or within the home.

The Ministry of Healing, 276.

EVERY form of uncleanliness tends to disease. Death-producing germs abound in dark, neglected corners, in decaying refuse, in dampness and mold and must. No waste vegetables or heaps of fallen leaves should be allowed to remain near the house, to decay and poison the air. Nothing unclean or decaying should be tolerated within the home. In towns or cities regarded perfectly healthful, many an epidemic of fever has been traced to decaying matter about the dwelling of some careless householder.

82. Drowsiness and dullness in church or school may be the result of improper ventilation.

The Ministry of Healing, 274.

IN THE construction of buildings, whether for public purposes or as dwellings, care should be taken to provide for good ventilation and plenty of sunlight. Churches and school-rooms are often faulty in this respect. Neglect of proper ventilation is responsible for much of the drowsiness and dullness that destroy the effect of many a sermon and make the teacher's work toilsome and ineffective.

83. Every room in the house, especially the bedrooms, should have a free circulation of air and plenty of sunlight.

The Ministry of Healing, 274.

IN THE building of houses it is especially important to secure thorough ventilation and plenty of sunlight. Let there be a current of air and an abundance of light in every room in the house. Sleeping rooms should be so arranged as to have a free circulation of air day and night. No room is fit to be occupied as a sleeping-room unless it can be thrown open daily to the air and sunshine. In most countries bedrooms need to be supplied with conveniences for heating, that they may be thoroughly warmed and dried in cold or wet weather.

84. The best conditions for house plants is also the most healthy for us.

The Ministry of Healing, 275.

IN BUILDING, many make careful provision for their plants and flowers. The greenhouse or window devoted to their use is warm and sunny; for without warmth, air, and sunshine, plants would not live and flourish. If these conditions are necessary to the life of plants, how much more necessary are they for our own health and that of our families and guests!.

85. The air in ill-ventilated rooms contains increased amounts of body wastes, the breathing of which weakens the entire system.

The Ministry of Healing, 274.

THE lungs are constantly throwing off impurities, and they need to be constantly supplied with fresh air. Impure air does not afford the necessary supply of oxygen, and the blood passes to the brain and other organs without being vitalized. Hence the necessity of thorough ventilation. To live in close, ill-ventilated rooms, where the air is dead and vitiated, weakens the entire system. It becomes peculiarly sensitive to the influence of cold, and a slight exposure induces disease. It is close confinement indoors that makes many women pale and feeble. They breathe the same air over and over, until it becomes laden with poisonous matter thrown off through the lungs and pores; and impurities are thus conveyed back to the blood.

86. The air in rooms without adequate ventilation and sunlight is unhealthy.

Counsels on Health, 57.

ROOMS that are not exposed to light and air become damp. Beds and bedding gather dampness, and the atmosphere in these rooms is poisonous, because it has not been purified by light and air.

87. Windows in bedrooms should be opened for several hours each day to let in fresh air and sun-

light.

Counsels on Health, 57.

SLEEPING rooms especially should be well ventilated, and the atmosphere made healthy by light and air. Blinds should be left open several hours each day, and the curtains put aside, and the rooms thoroughly aired. Nothing should remain, even for a short time, which would destroy the purity of the atmosphere.

88. Bedrooms need a free circulation of air day and night, winter and summer.

Counsels on Health, 57.

SLEEPING apartments should be large, and so arranged as to have a circulation of air through them day and night. Those who have excluded the air from their sleeping rooms, should begin to change their course immediately. They should let in air by degrees, and increase its circulation until they can bear it winter and summer, with no danger of taking cold. The lungs, in order to be healthy, must have pure air.

89. Pure air in the bedroom provides refreshing sleep at night and serves to remove the impurities from the exposed bed linens during the day.

Counsels on Health, 58.

THOSE who have not had a free circulation of air in their rooms through the night, generally awake feeling exhausted and feverish, and know not the cause. It was air, vital air, that the whole system required, but which it could not obtain. Upon rising in the morning, most persons would be benefited by taking a sponge bath, or, if more agreeable, a hand bath, with merely a washbowl of water. This will remove impurities from the skin. Then the clothing should be removed piece by piece from the bed, and exposed to the air. The windows should be opened, the blinds fastened back, and the air allowed to circulate freely for several hours, if not all day, through the sleeping apartments. In this manner the bed and clothing will become thoroughly aired, and the impurities will be removed from the room.

90. Bedrooms that are not exposed freely to the air and sunlight are a danger to health.

Counsels on Health, 57.

SOME houses are furnished expensively, more to gratify pride, and to receive visitors, than for the comfort, convenience, and health of the family. The best rooms are kept dark. The light and air are shut out, lest the light of heaven should injure the rich furniture, fade the carpets, or tarnish the picture frames. When visitors are seated in these rooms, they are in danger of taking cold, because of the cellarlike atmosphere pervading them. Parlor chambers and bedrooms are kept closed in the same manner and for the same reasons. And whoever occupies these beds which have not been freely exposed to light and air, do so at the expense of health, and often of life itself.

91. Bedrooms open to the fresh, outside air also need a source of heat in order to prevent the accumulation of moisture.

The Ministry of Healing, 275.

THE guest-chamber should have equal care with the rooms intended for constant use. Like the other bedrooms, it should have air and sunshine, and should be provided with some means of heating, to dry out the dampness that always accumulates in a room not in constant use. Whoever sleeps in a sunless room or occupies a bed that has not been thoroughly dried and aired, does so at the risk of health, and often of life.

92. The aged especially need to maintain their vigor by exposure to plenty of sunlight and fresh air.

The Ministry of Healing, 275.

THOSE who have the aged to provide for should remember that these especially need warm, comfortable rooms. Vigor declines as years advance, leaving less vitality with which to resist unhealthful influences; hence the greater necessity for the aged to have plenty of sunlight, and fresh, pure air.

93. For the sick, fresh air is more important than food; but they should not be placed in a draft.

Counsels on Health, 55.

IN NO case should sick persons be deprived of a full supply of fresh air in pleasant weather. Their rooms may not always be so constructed as to allow the windows or doors to be opened, without the draft coming directly upon them, thus exposing them to the taking of cold. In such cases windows and doors should be opened in an adjoining room, thus letting fresh air enter the room occupied by the sick. Fresh air will prove far more beneficial to sick persons than medicine, and is far more essential to them than their food. They will do better, and will recover sooner, when deprived of food, than when deprived of fresh air.

94. To avoid direct drafts, the sick, if necessary, should be temporarily moved to another room while their bed and bedding are aired out.

Counsels on Health, 56.

THE sick-room, if possible, should have a draft of air through it, day and night. The draft should not come directly upon the invalid. While burning fevers are raging, there is but little danger of taking cold. But special care is needful when the crisis comes, and the fever is passing away. Then constant watching may be necessary to keep vitality in the system. The sick must have pure, invigorating air. If no other way can be devised, the sick, if possible, should be removed to another room and another bed, while the sickroom, the bed and bedding are being purified by ventilation. If those who are well need the blessings of light and air, and need to observe habits of cleanliness in order to remain well, the need of the sick is still greater in proportion to their debilitated condition.

95. Many invalids fail to appreciate the value of sunlight and pure air.

Counsels on Health, 55.

MANY invalids have been confined for weeks and even for months in close rooms, with the light and the pure, invigorating air of heaven shut out, as if air were a deadly enemy, when it was just the medicine they needed to make them well. . . . These valuable remedies which Heaven has provided, without money and without price, were cast aside, and considered not only as worthless, but even as dangerous enemies, while poisons, prescribed by physicians, were in blind confidence taken.

96. Thousands have perished and other thousands have remained invalids from failure to use the benefits of pure air and the other natural remedies.

Counsels on Health, 55.

THOUSANDS have died for want of pure water, and pure air, who might have lived. And thousands of invalids, who are a burden to themselves and others, think that their lives depend upon taking medicines from the doctors. They are continually guarding themselves against the air, and avoiding the use of water. These blessings they need in order to become well. If they would become enlightened, and let medicine alone, and accustom themselves to outdoor exercise, and to air in their houses, summer and winter, and use soft water for drinking and bathing purposes, they would be comparatively well and happy, instead of dragging out a miserable existence.

97. If fresh air is not welcomed into the room of the sick, the attendants should fulfill their needs by getting exercise in the open air.

Counsels on Health, 56.

IT IS the duty of attendants and nurses to take special care of their own health, especially in critical cases of fever and consumption. One person should not be kept closely confined to the sick-room. It is safer to have two or three to depend upon, who are careful and understanding nurses, these changing and sharing the care and confinement of the sick-room. Each should have exercise in the open air, as often as possible. This is important to sick-bed attendants, especially if the friends of the sick are among the class that continue to regard air, if admitted into the sick-room, as an enemy, and will not allow the windows raised, or the doors opened. In such cases the sick and the attendants are compelled to breathe the poisonous atmosphere from day to day, because of the inexcusable ignorance of the friends of the sick.

98. Many attendants, because of their own ignorance of the importance of pure air in the sick-room, are likely to become ill.

Counsels on Health, 56.

IN VERY many cases the attendants are ignorant of the needs of the system, and of the relation that the breathing of fresh air sustains to health, and of the life-destroying influence of inhaling the impure air of a sick-room. In this case the life of the sick is endangered, and the attendants themselves are liable to take on disease, and lose health, and perhaps life.

99. Christ can best be presented to the sick while they are out-of-doors in the fresh air.

The Ministry of Healing, 266.

OUT-OF-DOORS, amid the things that God has made, breathing the fresh, health-giving air, the sick can best be told of the new life in Christ. Here God's Word can be read. Here the light of Christ's righteousness can shine into hearts darkened by sin.

100. The fragrance of certain trees, especially in association with the open air of the country, is health restoring.

The Ministry of Healing, 264.

PHYSICIANS and nurses should encourage their patients to be much in the open air. Outdoor life is the only remedy that many invalids need. It has a wonderful power to heal diseases caused by the excitements and excesses of fashionable life, a life that weakens and destroys the powers of body, mind, and soul. How grateful to the invalids weary of city life, the glare of many lights, and the noise of the streets, are the quiet and freedom of the country! How eagerly do they turn to the scenes of nature! How glad would they be to sit in the open air, rejoice in the sunshine, and breathe the fragrance of tree and flower! There are life-giving properties in the balsam of the pine, in the fragrance of the cedar and the fir, and other trees also have properties that are health-restoring.

101. The murmuring breezes assist nature in the restoration of the health of the chronic invalids.

The Ministry of Healing, 264.

TO THE chronic invalid, nothing so tends to restore health and happiness as living amid attractive country surroundings. Here the most helpless ones can sit or lie in the sunshine or in the shade of the trees. They have only to lift their eyes to see above them the beautiful foliage. A sweet sense of restfulness and refreshing comes over them as they listen to the murmuring of the breezes. The drooping spirits revive. The waning strength is recruited. Unconsciously the mind becomes peaceful, the fevered pulse more calm and regular. As the sick grow stronger, they will venture to take a few steps to gather some of the lovely flowers, precious messengers of God's love to His afflicted family here below.

102. Prescribed time in the open air, especially doing gardening, is beneficial to the sick.

The Ministry of Healing, 265.

EXERCISE in the open air should be prescribed as a life-giving necessity. And for such exercises there is nothing better than the cultivation of the soil. Let patients have flower beds to care for, or work to do in the orchard or vegetable garden. As they are encouraged to leave their rooms and spend time in the open air, cultivating flowers or doing some other light, pleasant work, their attention will be diverted from themselves and their sufferings.

103. The ill who are able to work should be provided outdoor labor and also be trained in how to breath.

The Ministry of Healing, 264.

PLANS should be devised for keeping patients out-of-doors. For those who are able to work, let some pleasant, easy employment be provided. Show them how agreeable and helpful this outdoor work is. Encourage them to breathe the fresh air. Teach them to breathe deeply, and in breathing and speaking to exercise the abdominal muscles. This is an education that will be invaluable to them.

104. Health-care institutions will be far more successful when located in the country amidst the pure air and the other physicians of nature.

The Ministry of Healing, 263–264.

INSTITUTIONS for the care of the sick would be far more successful if they could be established away from the cities. And so far as possible, all who are seeking to recover health should place themselves amid country surroundings, where they can have the benefit of outdoor life. Nature is God's physician. The pure air, the glad sunshine, the flowers and trees, the orchards and vineyards, and out-door exercise amid these surroundings, are health-giving, life-giving.

The True Remedies—II
Sunlight

See also paragraphs 79, 81–84, 86–87, 90–92, 94–95.

105. Sunlight is an integral part of the function and beauty of this earth.

Testimonies, vol. 5, 312.

HOW wonderfully, with what marvelous beauty, has everything in nature been fashioned. Everywhere we see the perfect works of the great Master Artist. The heavens declare His glory; and the earth, which is formed for the happiness of man, speaks to us of His matchless love. Its surface is not a monotonous plain, but grand old mountains rise to diversify the landscape. There are sparkling streams and fertile valleys, beautiful lakes, broad rivers, and the boundless ocean. God sends the dew and the rain to refresh the thirsty earth. The breezes, that promote health by purifying and cooling the atmosphere, are controlled by His wisdom. He has placed the sun in the heavens to mark the periods of day and night, and by its genial beams give light and warmth to the earth, causing vegetation to flourish.

106. God desires that His children live in harmony with the night and day cycles He has established.

Evangelism, 651.

SOME . . . are much opposed to order and discipline. They lie in bed some hours after daylight, when everyone should be astir. They burn the midnight oil, depending upon artificial light to supply the place of the light that nature has provided at seasonable hours. . . . Thus they are sleeping soundly when they should be awake with nature and the early-rising birds. The precious habits of order are broken; and the moments thus idled away in the early morning set things out of course for the whole day.

Our God is a God of order, and He desires that His children shall will to bring themselves into order, and under His discipline. Would it not be better, therefore, to break up this habit of turning night into day, and the fresh hours of the morning into night?

107. Early to bed and early to rise is essential to Christian healthful living.

Sons and Daughters of God, 171.

IF YOUNG men and women would grow up to the full stature of Christ Jesus, they must treat themselves intelligently. . . . Unhealthful habits of every order—late hours at night, late hours in bed in the morning, rapid eating are to be overcome. Masticate your food thoroughly. Let there be no hurried eating. Have your room well ventilated day and night, and perform useful physical labor. . . . By properly using our powers to their fullest extent in the most useful employment, by keeping every organ in health, by so preserving every organ that mind, sinew, and muscle shall work harmoniously, we may do the most precious service for God.

108. Out-of-doors in the sunlight is a must for health and happiness.

My Life Today, 138.

THERE are but few who realize that, in order to enjoy health and cheerfulness, they must have an abundance of sunlight, pure air, and physical exercise. We pity little children who are kept confined indoors when the sun is shining gloriously without. Clothe your boys and girls comfortably and properly. . . . Then let them go out and exercise in the open air, and live to enjoy health and happiness. The pale and sickly grain-blade that has struggled up out of the cold of early spring puts out the natural and healthy deep green after enjoying for a few days the health-and-life-giving rays of the sun. Go out into the light and warmth of the glorious sun. . . . and share with vegetation its life-giving, healing power.

109. Open air and sunlight help to counteract the effects of a wrong diet.

Temperance, 159.

THEY who work in the open air will feel less injury from the use of flesh meats than those of sedentary habits, for sun and air are great helps to digestion, and do much to counteract the effect of wrong habits of eating and drinking.

110. I must get all the sunlight possible in harmony with the prudent care of my body.

Medical Ministry, 230.

IN REGARD to that which we can do for ourselves: There is a point that requires careful, thoughtful consideration. I must become acquainted with myself. I must be a learner always as to how to take care of this building, the body God has given me, that I may preserve it in the very best condition of health. I must eat those things which will be for my very best good physically, and I must take special care to have my clothing such as will conduce to a healthful circulation of the blood. I must not deprive myself of exercise and air. I must get all the sunlight that it is possible for me to obtain. I must have wisdom to be a faithful guardian of my body.

111. Light, which God has pronounced good, should not be excluded from our homes.

My Life Today, 138.

WHEN God had made our world, and darkness was upon the face of the deep, he said, Let there be light, and there was light. And God saw the light that it was good. Shall we close our houses, and exclude from them the light which God has pronounced good?

112. Every room is to be furnished and adorned with sunlight.

My Life Today, 138.

NO ROOM in the house should be considered furnished and adorned without the cheering, enlivening light and sunshine, which are Heaven's own free gift to man.

113. Sunlight in the rooms will improve the physical and mental health of the children.

Healthful Living, 229.

IF THE windows were freed from blinds and heavy curtains, and the air and sun permitted to enter freely the darkened rooms, there would be seen a change for the better in the mental and physical health of the children. The pure air would have an invigorating influence upon them, and the sun that carries healing in its beams would soothe and cheer, and make them happy, joyous, and healthy.

114. The disease-causing impurities from mold and mildew can be prevented by the admission of sunshine and fresh air.

Healthful Living, 229.

THE confined air of unventilated rooms meets us with sickening odors of mildew and mold, and the impurities exhaled from its inmates. . . . The emanations from damp, moldy rooms and clothing are poisonous to the system. . . . If all would appreciate the sunshine, and expose every article of clothing to its drying, purifying rays, mildew and mold would be prevented. . . . This is the only way rooms can be kept from impurities. . . . Every room in our dwellings should be daily thrown open to the healthful rays of the sun, and the purifying air should be invited in. This will be a preventive of disease.

115. We must keep trees, vines, and curtains from blocking sunlight's entrance.

The Ministry of Healing, 275.

IF WE would have our homes the abiding-place of health and happiness, we must place them above the miasma and fog of the lowlands, and give free entrance to heaven's life-giving agencies. Dispense with heavy curtains, open the windows and the blinds, allow no vines, however beautiful, to shade the windows, and permit no trees to stand so near the house as to shut out the sunshine. The sunlight may fade the drapery and the carpets, and tarnish the picture-frames; but it will bring a healthy glow to the cheeks of the children.

116. Sunshine may fade the carpets, but it will add color to the cheeks.

Testimonies, vol. 2, 527.

IF YOU would have your homes sweet and inviting, make them bright with air and sunshine. Remove your heavy curtains, open the windows, throw back the blinds, and enjoy the rich sunlight, even if it be at the expense of the colors of your carpets. The precious sunlight may fade your carpets, but it will give a healthful color to the cheeks of your children. If you have God's presence, and possess earnest, loving hearts, a humble home, made bright with air and sunlight, and cheerful with the welcome of unselfish hospitality, will be to your family, and to the weary traveler, a heaven below.

117. The blessings from sunlight are symbolic of the blessings that should emanate from the Christian to those around them.

Our High Calling, 296.

IT IS the privilege of the Christian to connect with the Source of light, and through this living connection become the light of the world. Christ's true followers will walk in the light as He is in the light, and therefore they will not travel in an uncertain way, stumbling because they walk in darkness. The Great Teacher is impressing upon His hearers the blessing which they may be to the world, represented as the sun rising in the east, dispelling the mist and shadows of darkness. The dawn gives place to day. The sun, gilding, tinting, and then glorifying the heavens with its blaze of light is a symbol of the Christian life. As the light of the sun is light and life and blessing to all that live, so should Christians, by their good works, by their cheerfulness and courage, be the light of the world. As the light of the sun chases away the shades of night and pours its glories on valleys and hills, so will the Christian reflect the Sun of Righteousness which shines on him.

The True Remedies—III
Abstemiousness

118. Scripture says to drink "a little wine" for one's health.

1 Timothy 5:23.

DRINK no longer water, but use a little wine for thy stomach's sake and thine often infirmities.

119. The Bible does not teach the use of wine containing alcohol.

Healthful Living, 113.

THE Bible nowhere teaches the use of intoxicating wine, either as a beverage or as a symbol of the blood of Christ.

120. Paul instructed Timothy to use unfermented grape juice for his health.

The Signs of the Times, vol. 4, 58.

FERMENTED liquor confuses the senses and perverts the powers of the being. God is dishonored when men have not sufficient respect for themselves to practice strict temperance. Fermented wine is not a natural production. The Lord never made it, and with its production He has nothing to do. Paul advised Timothy to take a little wine for his stomach's sake and oft infirmities, but he meant the unfermented juice of the grape. He did not advise Timothy to take what the Lord had prohibited.

121. The wine produced miraculously by Christ at the wedding feast was unfermented.

The Signs of the Times, vol. 4, 58.

SOME who claim to be Christians feel at liberty to use intoxicating drink, and in this particular they claim to be in harmony with Christ. But Christ did not set the example they claim to imitate. Be assured that He did not make intoxicating wine on the occasion of His first miracle. He gave to those present a drink which it is safe to give to all humanity, the pure juice of the grape. Christ never placed a glass of fermented liquor to His lips or to the lips of His disciples. Drunkenness was rare in Palestine, but Christ looked down the ages, and saw in every generation what the use of wine would do for the users, therefore at this feast He set a right example.

122. The milder fermented beverages such as wine and cider lay the foundation for the stronger drinks, and they also can produce even greater and more perverse changes in the character and passions.

Healthful Living, 112.

PERSONS may become just as really intoxicated on wine and cider as on stronger drinks, and the worst kind of inebriation is produced by these so-called milder drinks. The passions are more perverse; the transformation of character is greater, more determined and obstinate. A few quarts of cider and sweet wine may awaken a taste for strong drinks, and many who have become confirmed drunkards have thus laid the foundation of the drinking habit. . . . Moderate drinking is the school in which men are receiving an education for the drunkard's career. The taste for stimulants is cultivated; the nervous system is disordered; Satan keeps the mind in a fever of unrest; and the poor victim, imagining himself perfectly secure, goes on and on, until every barrier is broken down, every principle sacrificed.

123. A single glass of wine can be the downfall of an individual.

Testimonies, vol. 4, 578.

WHEN there has been a departure from the right path, it is difficult to return. Barriers have been removed, safeguards broken down. One step in the wrong direction prepares the way for another. A single glass of wine may open the door of temptation which will lead to habits of drunkenness.

124. Total abstinence is the only platform on which to stand.

Testimonies, vol. 7, 75.

WHEN temperance is presented as a part of the gospel, many will see their need of reform. They will see the evil of intoxicating liquors and that total abstinence is the only platform on which God's people can conscientiously stand.

125. True temperance involves the proper use of even that which is healthful.

Patriarchs and Prophets, 562.

TRUE temperance teaches us to dispense entirely with everything hurtful, and to use judiciously that which is healthful.

126. The hurtful indulgence of normal desires is intemperance and is the major cause of illness.

Temperance, 137.

INTEMPERANCE, in the true sense of the word, is at the foundation of the larger share of the ills of life, and it annually destroys its tens of thousands. For intemperance is not limited to the use of intoxicating liquors; it has a broader meaning, and includes the hurtful indulgence of any appetite or passion.

127. The smoking of tobacco, a slow poison, is more addictive than alcohol, and it poisons the air that others breathe.

Christian Temperance and Bible Hygiene, 33–34.

WHEREVER we go, we encounter the tobacco devotee, enfeebling both mind and body by his darling indulgence. Have men a right to deprive their Maker and the world of the service which is their due? Tobacco is a slow, insidious poison. Its effects are more difficult to cleanse from the system than are those of liquor. It binds the victim in even stronger bands of slavery than does the intoxicating cup. It is a disgusting habit, defiling to the user, and very annoying to others. We rarely pass through a crowd but men will puff their poisoned breath in our faces. It is unpleasant, if not dangerous, to remain in a railway car or in a room where the atmosphere is impregnated with the fumes of liquor and tobacco. Is it honest thus to contaminate the air which others must breathe?

128. Infants especially are susceptible to the poisons given off by the breath and skin of the tobacco user.

Temperance, 58–59.

THE infant lungs suffer, and become diseased by inhaling the atmosphere of a room poisoned by the tobacco user's tainted breath. Many infants are poisoned beyond remedy by sleeping in beds with their tobacco-using fathers. By inhaling the poisonous tobacco effluvia, which is thrown from the lungs and pores of the skin, the system of the infant is filled with poison. While it acts upon some infants as a slow poison, it affects the brain, heart, liver, and lungs, and they waste away and fade gradually, upon others, it has a more direct influence, causing spasms, fits, paralysis, and sudden death.

129. True conversion liberates from health-destroying habits, and the users of alcohol and tobacco should manifest this liberty before they are baptized.

Evangelism, 264.

MEN and women have many habits that are antagonistic to the principles of the Bible. The victims of strong drink and tobacco are corrupted, body, soul, and spirit. Such ones should not be received into the church until they give evidence that they are truly converted, that they feel the need of the faith that works by love and purifies the soul. The truth of God will purify the true believer. He who is thoroughly converted will abandon every defiling habit and appetite. By total abstinence he will overcome his desire for health-destroying indulgences.

130. Tea and coffee, not being nutrients, stimulate a temporary, false energy, which is harmful rather than beneficial.

Testimonies, vol. 2, 65.

TEA and coffee do not nourish the system. The relief obtained from them is sudden, before the stomach has time to digest them. This shows that what the users of these stimulants call strength is only received by exciting the nerves of the stomach, which convey the irritation to the brain, and this in turn is aroused to impart increased action to the heart and short lived energy to the entire system. All this is false strength that we are the worse for having. They do not give a particle of natural strength.

131. The degree of stimulation above normal derived from tea and coffee use is followed by an equivalent prostration below normal.

Counsels on Diet and Foods, 421.

TEA is poisonous to the system. Christians should let it alone. The influence of coffee is in a degree the same as tea, but the effect upon the system is still worse. Its influence is exciting, and just in the degree that it elevates above par, it will exhaust and bring prostration below par.

132. Continued coffee use permanently lessens brain activity, leading to paralysis of the mental, moral, and physical powers.

Counsels on Diet and Foods, 421.

COFFEE is a hurtful indulgence. It temporarily excites the mind to unwonted action, but the aftereffect is exhaustion, prostration, paralysis of the mental, moral, and physical powers. The mind becomes enervated, and unless through determined effort the habit is overcome, the activity of the brain is permanently lessened.

133. The longevity of some who use these stimulants is not evidence that they escaped the enfeebling effects upon the body, especially those which war against spiritual progress.

Christian Temperance and Bible Hygiene, 34.

ALL these nerve irritants are wearing away the life forces, and the restlessness caused by shattered nerves, the mental feebleness, become a warring element, antagonizing to spiritual progress. Then should not those who advocate temperance and reform be awake to counteract the evils of these injurious drinks? In some cases it is as difficult to break up the tea-and-coffee habit as it is for the inebriate to discontinue the use of liquor. The money expended for tea and coffee is worse then wasted. They do the user only harm, and that continually. Those who use tea, coffee, opium, and alcohol, may sometimes live to old age, but this fact is no argument in favor of the use of these stimulants. What these persons might have accomplished, but failed to do because of their intemperate habits, the great day of God alone will reveal.

134. Given a chance, Nature will eventually overcome the withdrawal effects resulting from leaving off these unnatural stimulants.

Testimonies, vol. 1, 549.

THOSE who make a change and leave off these unnatural stimulants will for a time feel their loss and suffer considerably without them, as does the drunkard who is wedded to his liquor. Take away intoxicating drinks and he suffers terribly. But if he persists he will soon overcome the dreadful lack. Nature will come to his aid and remain at her post until he again substitutes the false prop in her place. Some have so benumbed the fine sensibilities of Nature that it may require a little time for her to recover from the abuse she has been made to suffer through the sinful habits of man, the indulgence of an acquired, depraved appetite, which has depressed and weakened her powers. Give Nature a chance, and she will rally and again perform her part nobly and well.

135. It is impossible for the users of unnatural stimulants to appreciate eternal values such as salvation which Christ's life of self-denial makes available.

Testimonies, vol. 1, 549.

THE use of unnatural stimulants is destructive to health and has a benumbing influence upon the brain, making it impossible to appreciate eternal things. Those who cherish these idols cannot rightly value the salvation which Christ has wrought out for them by a life of self-denial, continual suffering and reproach, and by finally yielding His own sinless life to save perishing man from death.

136. Tea, coffee, and flesh meats, through their stimulant effects, lead to a craving for stronger stimulants such as tobacco and alcohol.

Testimonies, vol. 3, 487–488.

INTEMPERANCE commences at our tables in the use of unhealthful food. After a time, through continued indulgence, the digestive organs become weakened, and the food taken does not satisfy the appetite. Unhealthy conditions are established, and there is craving for more stimulating food. Tea, coffee, and flesh meats produce an immediate effect. Under the influence of these poisons the nervous system is excited, and, in some cases, for the time being, the intellect seems to be invigorated and the imagination to be more vivid. Because these stimulants produce for the time being such agreeable results, many conclude that they really need them and continue their use. But there is always a reaction. The nervous system, having been unduly excited, borrowed power for present use from its future resources of strength. All this temporary invigoration of the system is followed by depression. In proportion as these stimulants temporarily invigorate the system will be the letting down of the power of the excited organs after the stimulus has lost its force. The appetite is educated to crave something stronger which will have a tendency to keep up and increase the agreeable excitement, until indulgence becomes habit, and there is a continual craving for stronger stimulus, as tobacco, wines, and liquors. The more the appetite is indulged, the more frequent will be its demands and the more difficult of control. The more debilitated the system becomes and the less able to do without unnatural stimulus, the more the passion for these things increases, until the will is over borne, and there seems to be no power to deny the unnatural craving for these indulgences.

137. Rich, highly seasoned foods and also flesh foods excite a desire for the stimulating drinks.

Counsels on Diet and Foods, 268–269.

THE food is often such as to excite a desire for stimulating drinks. Luxurious dishes are placed before the children, spiced foods, rich gravies, cakes, and pastries. This highly seasoned food irritates the stomach, and causes a craving for the use of these many harmful substances. When the message comes to those who have not heard the truth for this time, they see that a great reformation must take place in their diet. They see that they must put away flesh food, because it creates an appetite for liquor, and fills the system with disease.

138. Parents that indulge their children with tea, coffee, and flesh meats are forming the appetites for the nerve debilitating use of tobacco and liquor.

Testimonies, vol. 3, 488–489.

MANY parents educate the tastes of their children and form their appetites. They indulge them in eating flesh meats and in drinking tea and coffee. The highly seasoned flesh meats and the tea and coffee, which some mothers encourage their children to use, prepare the way for them to crave stronger stimulants, as tobacco. The use of tobacco encourages the appetite for liquor, and the use of tobacco and liquor invariably lessens nerve power.

139. Total abstinence from stimulants is the only safe course.

Testimonies, vol. 3, 488.

THE only safe course is to touch not, taste not, handle not, tea, coffee, wines, tobacco, opium, and alcoholic drinks.

140. Pure water is the only beverage that nature requires.

Temperance, 101.

IF ANYTHING is needed to quench thirst, pure water drunk some little time before or after the meal is all that nature requires. Never take tea, coffee, beer, wine, or any spirituous liquors. Water is the best liquid possible to cleanse the tissues.

141. True temperance not only abstains from intoxicating liquors and tobacco, but regulates the diet as well.

Counsels on Diet and Foods, 406.

WE ARE health reformers, seeking to come back, as far as possible, to the Lord's original plan of temperance. Temperance does not consist merely in abstaining from intoxicating liquors and tobacco; it extends farther than this. It must regulate what we eat.

142. True temperance involves subjecting the bodily appetites to the intellectual powers of the mind.

Patriarchs and Prophets, 562.

THE principles of temperance must be carried further than the mere use of spirituous liquors. The use of stimulating and indigestible food is often equally injurious to health, and in many cases sows the seeds of drunkenness. True temperance teaches us to dispense entirely with everything hurtful and to use judiciously that which is healthful. There are few who realize as they should how much their habits of diet have to do with their health, their character, their usefulness in this world, and their eternal destiny. The appetite should ever be in subjection to the moral and intellectual powers. The body should be servant to the mind, and not the mind to the body.

143. Intemperance, even in eating healthful food, lies at the foundation of the mental and physical feebleness apparent everywhere.

Testimonies, vol. 3, 487.

INTEMPERANCE in eating, even of food of the right quality, will have a prostrating influence upon the system and will blunt the keener and holier emotions. Strict temperance in eating and drinking is highly essential for the healthy preservation and vigorous exercise of all the functions of the body. Strictly temperate habits, combined with exercise of the muscles as well as of the mind, will preserve both mental and physical vigor, and give power of endurance to those engaged in the ministry, to editors, and to all others whose habits are sedentary. As a people, with all our profession of health reform, we eat too much. Indulgence of appetite is the greatest cause of physical and mental debility, and lies at the foundation of the feebleness which is apparent everywhere.

144. Intemperate eating frequently causes sickness, which generally will respond to dietary abstemiousness.

The Ministry of Healing, 235.

INTEMPERATE eating is often the cause of sickness, and what nature most needs is to be relieved of the undue burden that has been placed upon her. In many cases of sickness, the very best remedy is for the patient to fast for a meal or two, that the overworked organs of digestion may have an opportunity to rest. A fruit diet for a few days has often brought great relief to brain workers. Many times a short period of entire abstinence from food, followed by simple, moderate eating, has led to recovery through nature's own recuperative effort. An abstemious diet for a month or two would convince many sufferers that the path of self-denial is the path to health.

145. Abstemiousness in diet improves mental and moral vigor, which is especially beneficial to those with a sluggish temperament.

The Ministry of Healing, 308.

ABSTEMIOUSNESS in diet is rewarded with mental and moral vigor; it also aids in the control of the passions. Overeating is especially harmful to those who are sluggish in temperament; these should eat sparingly and take plenty of physical exercise. There are men and women of excellent natural ability who do not accomplish half what they might if they would exercise self-control in the denial of appetite.

146. Control of appetite is essential to Christian perfection.

Christian Temperance and Bible Hygiene, 37.

IT IS impossible for those who give the reins to appetite to attain to Christian perfection.

147. Christ fasted forty days in order to set us an example and to reveal the importance of and the serious struggle required to overcome the indulgence of appetite.

Testimonies, vol. 3, 486.

THE Redeemer of the world knew that the indulgence of appetite would bring physical debility, and so deaden the perceptive organs that sacred and eternal things would not be discerned. Christ knew that the world was given up to gluttony and that this indulgence would pervert the moral powers. If the indulgence of appetite was so strong upon the race that, in order to break its power, the divine Son of God, in behalf of man, was required to fast nearly six weeks, what a work is before the Christian in order that he may overcome even as Christ overcame! The strength of the temptation to indulge perverted appetite can be measured only by the inexpressible anguish of Christ in that long fast in the wilderness.

148. We need even more power from God than previous generations to overcome perverted appetite, and only thus can we prevent Satan from controlling us mind and body.

Christian Temperance and Bible Hygiene, 37.

THROUGH appetite, Satan controls the mind and the whole being. Thousands who might have lived, have passed into the grave, physical, mental, and moral wrecks, because they sacrificed all their powers to the indulgence of appetite. The necessity for the men of this generation to call to their aid the power of the will, strengthened by the grace of God, in order to with stand the perverted appetite, is far greater than it was several generations ago. But the present generation have less power of self-control than had those who lived then. Those who indulged in these stimulants transmitted their depraved appetites and passions to their children, and greater moral power is now required to resist intemperance in all its forms. The only perfectly safe course is to stand firm, observing strict temperance in all things, and never venturing into the path of danger.

149. Christ came to teach us the necessity of self-denial, and also to bring us power to overcome appetite and thus to be victors on every point.

Testimonies, vol. 3, 488.

THE great end for which Christ endured that long fast in the wilderness was to teach us the necessity of self-denial and temperance. This work should commence at our tables and should be strictly carried out in all the concerns of life. The Redeemer of the world came from heaven to help man in his weakness, that, in the power which Jesus came to bring him, he might become strong to overcome appetite and passion, and might be victor on every point.

150. Only the Bible can teach us true temperance, and the example of Daniel and his associates is the most forcible example.

Christian Temperance and Bible Hygiene, 25.

IN ORDER rightly to understand the subject of temperance, we must consider it from a Bible standpoint; and nowhere can we find a more comprehensive and forcible illustration of true temperance and its attendant blessings, than is afforded by the history of the prophet Daniel and his Hebrew associates in the court of Babylon.

151. Obedience to natural law honored the Hebrew captives with unrivaled physical and mental health.

Christian Temperance and Bible Hygiene, 27.

GOD always honors the right. The most promising youth from all the lands subdued by the great conqueror had been gathered at Babylon, yet amid them all, the Hebrew captives were without a rival. The erect form, the firm, elastic step, the fair countenance, the undimmed senses, the untainted breath, all were so many certificates of good habits insignia of the nobility with which nature honors those who are obedient to her laws.

152. The noble witness for true temperance by Daniel and his companions may be repeated by the youth of today.

Christian Temperance and Bible Hygiene, 27.

THE history of Daniel and his companions has been recorded on the pages of the inspired word, for the benefit of the youth of all succeeding ages. What men have done, men may do. Did those youthful Hebrews stand firm amid great temptations, and bear a noble testimony in favor of true temperance? the youth of to-day may bear a similar testimony.

153. As a child, John the Baptist was raised with strictly temperate habits, to prepare him for the work of reform to prepare the way for Christ.

Counsels on Diet and Foods, 225.

ABOUT the time of Christ's first advent the angel Gabriel came to Zacharias with a message similar to that given to Manoah. The aged priest was told that his wife should bear a son, whose name should be called John. "And," said the angel, "thou shalt have joy and gladness; and many shall rejoice at his birth. For he shall be great in the sight of the Lord, and shall drink neither wine nor strong drink; and he shall be filled with the Holy Ghost." This child of promise was to be brought up with strictly temperate habits. An important work of reform was to be committed to him, to prepare the way for Christ.

154. John's example and message was to rebuke the debilitating indulgence of appetite prevalent in his day.

Counsels on Diet and Foods, 40.

INTEMPERANCE in every form existed among the people. Indulgence in wine and luxurious food was lessening physical strength, and debasing the morals to such an extent that the most revolting crimes did not appear sinful. The voice of John was to sound forth from the wilderness in stern rebuke for the sinful indulgences of the people, and his own abstemious habits were also to be a reproof of the excesses of his time.

155. Abstinence from harmful substances is the only way to prevent ruin of mind and body.

Medical Ministry, 221.

THE distinction between prevention and cure has not been made sufficiently important. Teach the people that it is better to know how to keep well than how to cure disease. Our physicians should be wise educators, warning all against self-indulgence, showing that abstinence from the things that God has prohibited is the only way to prevent ruin of body and mind.

156. Our health institutions should instruct their patients in the blessing of total abstinence from alcohol and an abundance of fruit should be provided to take its place.

Counsels on Diet and Foods, 311.

IN OUR medical institutions clear instruction should be given in regard to temperance. The patients should be shown the evil of intoxicating liquor, and the blessing of total abstinence. They should be asked to discard the things that have ruined their health, and the place of these things should be supplied with an abundance of fruit. Oranges, lemons, prunes, peaches, and many other varieties can be obtained; for the Lord's world is productive, if painstaking effort is put forth.

157. We are to press home total abstinence from alcohol and tobacco with all the force of the Holy Spirit's unction.

Evangelism, 534.

PRESS home the temperance question with all the force of the Holy Spirit's unction. Show the need of total abstinence from all intoxicating liquor. Show the terrible harm that is wrought in the human system by the use of tobacco and alcohol. Explain your methods of giving treatment. Let the talks given be such as will enlighten your hearers. God has mercy on the unrighteous. This service will be an opportunity to tell what health reform really is.

158. Many of the higher classes will accept the principles of true temperance when they are presented in the light of the plan of salvation.

The Ministry of Healing, 211.

THOUSANDS in positions of trust and honor are indulging habits that mean ruin to soul and body. Ministers of the gospel, statesmen, authors, men of wealth and talent, men of vast business capacity and power for usefulness, are in deadly peril because they do not see the necessity of self-control in all things. They need to have their attention called to the principles of temperance, not in a narrow or arbitrary way, but in the light of God's great purpose for humanity. Could the principles of true temperance thus be brought before them, there are very many of the higher classes who would recognize their value and give them a hearty acceptance.

159. Not many of the higher classes will refuse to listen when total abstinence is presented in its full light.

The Ministry of Healing, 211.

WE SHOULD show these persons the result of harmful indulgences in lessening physical, mental, and moral power. Help them to realize their responsibility as stewards of God's gifts. Show them the good they could do with the money they now spend for that which does them only harm. Present the total abstinence pledge, asking that the money they would otherwise spend for liquor, tobacco, or like indulgences work be devoted to the relief of the sick poor or for the training of children and youth for usefulness in the world. To such an appeal not many would refuse to listen.

160. We are to teach that alcoholism is not only a physical disease; but also a moral sin, and that the only solution is through total abstinence by the power of God.

Healthful Living, 114.

WHAT cure would you advise for a person who thus indulges a habit that is rebuked even by the beasts of the field? The word of God has denounced it: no drunkard shall enter the kingdom of God. What would you recommend to cure such an appetite? You would not say, "You may use strong drink moderately. Continue within bounds, but never indulge to excess." You would rather say, "There is no such thing as helping you unless you cooperate fully with my efforts, and sign the pledge of total abstinence. You have by indulgence made your habit second nature, and it cannot be controlled unless the moral power shall be aroused, and you look unto Jesus, trusting in the grace he shall give to overcome this unnatural craving." You would say, "You have lost your self-control. Your self-indulgence is not only a moral sin, but it has become a physical disease. You are not your own; with an infinite price, and every faculty is to be employed in his service. Keep your body in a healthy condition to do his will; keep your intellect clear and active to think candidly and critically, and to control all your powers."

161. The prosperity of a nation depends upon the strict temperance of its people.

Gospel Workers, 388.

THE prosperity of a nation is dependent upon the virtue and intelligence of its citizens. To secure these blessings, habits of strict temperance are indispensable. The history of ancient kingdoms is replete with lessons of warning for us. Luxury, self-indulgence, and dissipation prepared the way for their downfall. It remains to be seen whether our own republic will be admonished by their example, and avoid their fate.

162. The accusing conscience of those indulging appetite is injured when straight truth is spoken, and this leads them, unless the fleshly lusts are crucified, to stand under the black banner of Satan.

Testimonies, vol. 1, 548.

SOME are indulging lustful appetite which wars against the soul and is a constant hindrance to their spiritual advancement. They constantly bear an accusing conscience, and if straight truths are talked they are prepared to be offended. They are self-condemned and feel that subjects have been purposely selected to touch their case. They feel grieved and injured, and withdraw themselves from the assemblies of the saints. They forsake the assembling of themselves together, for then their consciences are not so disturbed. They soon lose their interest in the meetings and their love for the truth, and, unless they entirely reform, will go back and take their position with the rebel host who stand under the black banner of Satan. If these will crucify fleshly lusts which war against the soul, they will get out of the way, where the arrows of truth will pass harmlessly by them. But while they indulge lustful appetite, and thus cherish their idols, they make themselves a mark for the arrows of truth to hit, and if truth is spoken at all, they must be wounded. Some think that they cannot reform, that health would be sacrificed should they attempt to leave the use of tea, tobacco, and flesh meats. This is the suggestion of Satan. It is these hurtful stimulants that are surely undermining the constitution and preparing the system for acute diseases by impairing Nature's fine machinery; and battering down her fortifications erected against disease and premature decay.

163. True religion leads to victory over all health-destroying indulgences.

Testimonies, vol. 9, 113.

ABSTINENCE from all hurtful food and drink is the fruit of true religion. He who is thoroughly converted will abandon every injurious habit and appetite. By total abstinence he will overcome his desire for health-destroying indulgences.

164. Strict temperance will guard us from even the excess use of God's bounties.

Christian Temperance and Bible Hygiene, 27.

OUR danger is not from scarcity, but from abundance. We are constantly tempted to excess. Those who would preserve their powers unimpaired for the service of God, must observe strict temperance in the use of his bounties, as well as total abstinence from every injurious or debasing indulgence.

The True Remedies—IV
Rest

165. Sleep restores, invigorates, and prepares the body for the next day's duties.

The Adventist Home, 289.

SLEEP, nature's sweet restorer, invigorates the weary body and prepares it for the next day's duties.

166. Since restoration of the body takes place during rest, regularity in rest is essential, especially for the youth.

Education, 205.

THE importance of regularity in the time for eating and sleeping should not be overlooked. Since the work of building up the body takes place during the hours of rest, it is essential, especially in youth, that sleep should be regular and abundant.

167. Those who are cheerful-minded, diligent workers have unbroken slumber at night.

Testimonies, vol. 2, 529.

THOSE who are always busy, and go cheerfully about the performance of their daily tasks, are the most happy and healthy. The rest and composure of night brings to their wearied frames unbroken slumber.

168. The custom of turning day into night and night into day is contrary to nature and order.

Child Guidance, 111–112.

HOW prevalent is the habit of turning day into night, and night into day. Many youth sleep soundly in the morning, when they should be up with the early singing birds and be stirring when all nature is awake.

Some youth are much opposed to order and discipline. They do not respect the rules of the home by rising at a regular hour. They lie in bed some hours after daylight, when everyone should be astir. They burn the midnight oil, depending upon artificial light to supply the place of the light that nature has provided at seasonable hours. In so doing they not only waste precious opportunities, but cause additional expense. But in almost every case the plea is made, "I cannot get through my work; I have something to do; I cannot retire early." . . . The precious habits of order are broken, and the moments thus idled away in the early morning set things out of course for the whole day.

169. Late meals, preventing rest of the digestive system during the night, causes irritability of the person, who then casts a shadow wherever he or she goes.

Counsels on Health, 118–119.

MANY indulge in the pernicious habit of eating just before retiring. They may have taken their regular meals, yet because they feel a sense of faintness, they think they must have a lunch. By indulging this wrong practice it becomes a habit, and they feel as though they could not sleep without food. In many cases this faintness comes because the digestive organs have been too severely taxed through the day in disposing of the great quantity of food forced upon them. These organs need a period of entire rest from labor, to recover their exhausted energies. A second meal should never be eaten until the stomach has had time to recover from labor of digesting the preceding meal. When we lie down at night, the stomach should have its work all done, that it, as well as other portions of the body, may enjoy rest. But if more food is forced upon it, the digestive organs are put in motion again, to perform the same round of labor through the sleeping hours. The sleep of such is often disturbed with unpleasant dreams, and in the morning they awake unrefreshed. When this practice is followed, the digestive organs lose their natural vigor, and the person finds himself a miserable dyspeptic. And not only does the transgression of nature's laws affect the individual unfavorably, but others suffer more or less with him. Let anyone take a course that irritates him in anyway, and see how quickly he manifests impatience. He cannot, without special grace, speak or act calmly. He casts a shadow wherever he goes. How can anyone say, then, "It is nobody's business what I eat or drink?".

170. The use of nerve stimulants leads to wakefulness, thus preventing the rest that the tired nervous system actually needs.

The Ministry of Healing, 326–327.

THE continued use of these nerve irritants is followed by headache, wakefulness, palpitation of the heart, indigestion, trembling, and many other evils; for they wear away the life forces. Tired nerves need rest and quiet instead of stimulation and overwork. Nature needs time to recuperate her exhausted energies. When her forces are goaded on by the use of stimulants, more will be accomplished for a time; but, as the system becomes debilitated by their continued use, it gradually becomes more difficult to rouse the energies to the desired point. The demand for stimulants becomes more difficult to control, until the will is overborne, and there seems to be no power to deny the unnatural craving. Stronger and still stronger stimulants are called for, until exhausted nature can no longer respond.

171. A clear conscience and perfect trust in God result in rest that invigorates and renews.

The Spirit of Prophecy, vol. 3, 338–339.

ON THIS last night before the execution a mighty angel, commissioned from heaven, descended to rescue him. The strong gates which shut in the saint of God open without the aid of human hands; the angel of the Most High enters, and they close again noiselessly behind him. He enters the cell, hewn from the solid rock, and there lies Peter, sleeping the blessed, peaceful sleep of innocence and perfect trust in God, while chained to a powerful guard on either side of him. The light which envelopes the angel illuminates the prison, but does not waken the sleeping apostle. His is the sound repose that invigorates and renews and that comes of a good conscience.

172. Dreams can be from the Lord or from Satan, but the vast majority are from the common things of life.

Testimonies, vol. 1, 569–570.

THE multitude of dreams arise from the common things of life, with which the Spirit of God has nothing to do. There are also false dreams, as well as false visions, which are inspired by the spirit of Satan. But dreams from the Lord are classed in the Word of God with visions and are as truly the fruits of the spirit of prophecy as visions. Such dreams, taking into the account the persons who have them and the circumstances under which they are given, contain their own proofs of their genuineness.

173. Clean and neat sleeping rooms help children's thoughts to be pure.

Counsels on Health, 103.

MOTHERS, if you desire your children's thoughts to be pure, let their surroundings be pure. Let their sleeping rooms be scrupulously neat and clean. Teach them to care for their clothing. Each child should have a place of his own to care for his clothes. Few parents are so poor that they can not afford to provide for this purpose a large box, which may be fitted with shelves and tastefully covered.

174. The Sabbath should not be used for rest, to make up for inadequate rest due to intemperance in work the other days of the week.

Testimonies, vol. 2, 704.

NONE should feel at liberty to spend sanctified time in an unprofitable manner. It is displeasing to God for Sabbathkeepers to sleep during much of the Sabbath. They dishonor their Creator in so doing, and by their example, say that the six days are too precious for them to spend in resting. They must make money, although it be by robbing themselves of needed sleep, which they make up by sleeping away holy time. They then excuse themselves by saying: "The Sabbath was given for a day of rest. I will not deprive myself of rest to attend meeting, for I need rest." Such make a wrong use of the sanctified day. They should, upon that day especially, interest their families in its observance and assemble at the house of prayer with the few or with the many, as the case may be. They should devote their time and energies to spiritual exercises, that the divine influence resting upon the Sabbath may attend them through the week. Of all the days in the week, none are so favorable for devotional thoughts and feelings as the Sabbath.

175. Proper forms of recreation are needed by both physical and mental laborers.

Testimonies, vol. 1, 514.

I WAS shown that Sabbathkeepers as a people labor too hard without allowing themselves change or periods of rest. Recreation is needful to those who are engaged in physical labor and is still more essential for those whose labor is principally mental. It is not essential to our salvation, nor for the glory of God, to keep the mind laboring constantly and excessively, even upon religious themes. There are amusements, such as dancing, card playing, chess, checkers, etc., which we cannot approve because Heaven condemns them. These amusements open the door for great evil. They are not beneficial in their tendency, but have an exciting influence, producing in some minds a passion for those plays which lead to gambling and dissipation. All such plays should be condemned by Christians, and something perfectly harmless should be substituted in their place.

176. Rather than scenes of senseless mirth, we need innocent recreation that better qualifies us to carry out our Christian duties.

Messages to Young People, 364.

IT IS the privilege and duty of Christians to seek to refresh their spirits and invigorate their bodies by innocent recreation, with the purpose of using their physical and mental powers to the glory of God. Our recreations should not be scenes of senseless mirth, taking the form of the nonsensical. We can conduct them in such a manner as will benefit and elevate those with whom we associate, and better qualify us and them to more successfully attend to the duties devolving upon us as Christians.

177. Contemplation of the works of God in nature is a form of recreation that is highly beneficial to both mind and body.

Testimonies, vol. 4, 653.

THERE are modes of recreation which are highly beneficial to both mind and body. An enlightened, discriminating mind will find abundant means for entertainment and diversion, from sources not only innocent, but instructive. Recreation in the open air, the contemplation of the works of God in nature, will be of the highest benefit.

178. True recreation gives vigor for the work of life, while amusement is a hindrance to success.

Education, 205.

THERE is a distinction between recreation and amusement. Recreation, when true to its name, re-creation, tends to strengthen and build up. Calling us aside from our ordinary cares and occupations, it affords refreshment for mind and body, and thus enables us to return with new vigor to the earnest work of life. Amusement, on the other hand, is sought for the sake of pleasure, and is often carried to excess; it absorbs the energies that are required for useful work, and thus proves a hindrance to life's true success.

179. The best form of recreation for children is some line of useful effort.

Education, 215.

AS A rule, the exercise most beneficial to the youth will be found in useful employment. The little child finds both diversion and development in play; and his sports should be such as to promote not only physical, but mental and spiritual growth. As he gains strength and intelligence, the best recreation will be found in some line of effort that is useful.

180. The sleep of children is sweet and refreshing after useful labor.

The Adventist Home, 289.

CHILDREN need more frequent change of employment and intervals of rest than grown persons do; but even when quite young, they may begin learning to work, and they will be happy in the thought that they are making themselves useful. Their sleep will be sweet after healthful labor, and they will be refreshed for the next day's work.

181. Holiday group excursions into nature with parents being children with their children will be physically and mentally beneficial to all.

Testimonies, vol. 1, 514–515.

I SAW that our holidays should not be spent in patterning after the world, yet they should not be passed by unnoticed, for this will bring dissatisfaction to our children. On these days when there is danger that our children will be exposed to evil influences, and become corrupted by the pleasures and excitement of the world, let the parents study to get up something to take the place of more dangerous amusements. Give your children to understand that you have their good and happiness in view.

Let several families living in a city or village unite and leave the occupations which have taxed them physically and mentally, and make an excursion into the country to the side of a fine lake or to a nice grove where the scenery of nature is beautiful. They should provide themselves with plain, hygienic food, the very best fruits and grains, and spread their table under the shade of some tree or under the canopy of heaven. The ride, the exercise, and the scenery will quicken the appetite, and they can enjoy a repast which kings might envy.

On such occasions parents and children should feel free from care, labor, and perplexity. Parents should become children with their children, making everything as pleasant for them as possible. Let the whole day be given to recreation. Exercise in the open air for those whose employment has been withindoors and sedentary will be beneficial to health. All who can, should feel it a duty to pursue this course. Nothing will be lost, but much gained. They can return to their occupations with new life and new courage to engage in their labors with zeal, and they are better prepared to resist disease.

182. The redeemed will experience physical, emotional, and spiritual rest.

My Life Today, 358.

THERE certainly is and ever will be employment in heaven. The whole family of the redeemed will not live in a state of dreamy idleness. There remaineth a rest to the people of God. In heaven activity will not be wearing and burdensome; it will be rest. The whole family of the redeemed will find their delight in serving Him whose they are by creation and by redemption. To the weary and heavy laden, to those who have fought the good fight of faith, it will be a glorious rest; for the youth and vigor of immortality will be theirs, and against sin and Satan they will no longer have to contend.

The True Remedies—V
Exercise

183. Man was designed for garden work in the open air.

Christian Temperance and Bible Hygiene, 172.

MAN'S employment, as seen in the original design is also worthy of notice. "The Lord God took the man, and put him into the garden of Eden to dress it and to keep it." Man was designed for activity in the open light of the sun and the free air of heaven. These conditions were important to the joys of his existence. The subsequent curse upon Adam was not in that he should labor, but that his labors should be attended with difficulties.

184. Man's organs were designed for labor, and no sooner did God create man than He gave him his appointed work.

Testimonies, vol. 3, 76.

GOD made Adam and Eve in Paradise, and surrounded them with everything that was useful and lovely. He planted for them a beautiful garden. No herb nor flower nor tree was wanting which might be for use or ornament. The Creator of man knew that the workmanship of His hands could not be happy without employment. Paradise delighted their souls, but this was not enough; they must have labor to call into exercise the wonderful organs of the body. The Lord had made the organs for use. Had happiness consisted in doing nothing, man, in his state of holy innocence, would have been left unemployed. But He who formed man knew what would be for his best happiness, and He no sooner made him than He gave him his appointed work. In order to be happy, he must labor.

185. A short period of trial will convince you of the many benefits of daily exercise in the open air.

Testimonies, vol. 2, 533.

THOSE who do not use their limbs every day will realize a weakness when they do attempt to exercise. The veins and muscles are not in a condition to perform their work and keep all the living machinery in healthful action, each organ in the system doing its part. The limbs will impart strength to the muscles, which without exercise become flabby and enfeebled. By active exercise in the open air every day, the liver, kidneys, and lungs also will be strengthened to perform their work. Bring to your aid the power of the will, which will resist cold and will give energy to the nervous system. In a short time you will so realize the benefit of exercise and pure air that you would not live without these blessings.

186. The blessings from daily labor and those from the plan of salvation were planned by the same Creator.

My Life Today, 168.

RICHES and idleness are thought by some to be blessings indeed; but those who are always busy, and who cheerfully go about their daily tasks, are the most happy and enjoy the best health. The healthful weariness which results from well-regulated labor secures to them the benefits of refreshing sleep. The sentence that man must toil for his daily bread, and the promise of future happiness and glory, both came from the same throne, and both are blessings.

187. Daily activity preserves the living machinery.

Healthful Living, 131.

GOD designed that the living machinery should be in daily activity; for in this activity or motion is its preserving power.

188. The harmonious action of the many components of the human body requires that they each be exercised regularly.

Testimonies, vol. 3, 77.

EACH faculty of the mind and each muscle has its distinctive office, and all require to be exercised in order to become properly developed and retain healthful vigor. Each organ and muscle has its work to do in the living organism. Every wheel in the machinery must be a living, active, working wheel. Nature's fine and wonderful works need to be kept in active motion in order to accomplish the object for which they were designed. Each faculty has a bearing upon the others, and all need to be exercised in order to be properly developed. If one muscle of the body is exercised more than another, the one used will become much the larger, and will destroy the harmony and beauty of the development of the system. A variety of exercise will call into use all the muscles of the body.

189. The mind will gain strength and knowledge by the harmonious exercise of the other organs.

Testimonies, vol. 3, 77.

GOD has given us all something to do. In the discharge of the various duties which we are to perform, which lie in our pathway, our lives will be made useful, and we shall be blessed. Not only will the organs of the body be strengthened by exercise, but the mind also will acquire strength and knowledge through the action of those organs. The exercise of one muscle, while others are left with nothing to do, will not strengthen the inactive ones any more than the continual exercise of one of the organs of the mind will develop and strengthen the organs not brought into use.

190. Ministers would have better health if they would intelligently exercise both mind and body.

Healthful Living, 132.

IF THEY worked intelligently, giving both mind and body a due share of exercise, ministers would not so readily succumb to disease.

191. When young, we need to learn balance between the exercise of the mind and of the body.

Healthful Living, 127.

THE human body may be compared to nicely adjusted machinery, which needs care to keep it in running order. One part should not be subjected to constant wear and pressure, while another part is rusting from inaction. While the mind is taxed, the muscles also should have their proportion of exercise. Every young person should learn how many hours may be spent in study, and how much time should be given to physical exercise.

192. An unbalanced mind can be prevented by varying the subject of thought and by balanced physical and mental exercise.

Education, 209.

BY PURSUING one line of thought exclusively, the mind often becomes unbalanced. But every faculty may be safely exercised if the mental and physical powers are equally taxed and the subjects of thought are varied.

193. Students who neglect physical exercise have a hot head and cold feet, which lead to poor health.

Healthful Living, 134.

IN WHAT contrast to the habits of the active farmer are those of the student who neglects physical exercise. . . . His blood moves sluggishly; his feet are cold; his head hot. How can such a person have health?

194. Physical exercise improves the circulation and thus invigorates the whole body.

Testimonies, vol. 3, 490.

IF PHYSICAL exercise were combined with mental exertion, the blood would be quickened in its circulation, the action of the heart would be more perfect, impure matter would be thrown off, and new life and vigor would be experienced in every part of the body.

195. Equalization of the circulation through exercise benefits every organ.

Healthful Living, 132.

THE proper use of their physical strength, as well as of the mental powers, will equalize the circulation of the blood, and keep every organ of the living machinery in running order.

196. Equalized circulation through useful employment invigorates the system to overcome bad conditions.

Healthful Living, 134.

USEFUL employment would bring into exercise the enfeebled muscles, enliven the stagnant blood in the system, and arouse the torpid liver to perform its work. The circulation of the blood would be equalized, and the entire system invigorated to overcome bad conditions.

197. Walking in the open air is the best means to preserve health, and one of the most efficient ways to recover health.

Healthful Living, 130.

THERE is no exercise that will prove as beneficial to every part of the body as walking. Active walking in the open air will do more for women, to preserve them in health if they are well, than any other means. Walking is also one of the most efficient remedies for the recovery of health of the invalid. The hands and arms are exercised as well as the limbs.

198. Those with diseased bodies, where possible, should walk; for there is no better exercise to improve the circulation.

Testimonies, vol. 3, 78.

WALKING in all cases where it is possible, is the best remedy for diseased bodies, because in this exercise all the organs of the body are brought into use. Many who depend upon the movement cure could accomplish more for themselves by muscular exercise than the movements can do for them. In some cases want of exercise causes the bowels and muscles to become enfeebled and shrunken, and these organs that have become enfeebled for want of use will be strengthened by exercise. There is no exercise that can take the place of walking. By it the circulation of the blood is greatly improved.

199. Gardening for exercise is just as much the work of God as is the holding of meetings.

Healthful Living, 129.

BRETHREN, when you take time to cultivate your gardens, thus gaining the exercise needed to keep the system in good working order, you are just as much doing the work of God as in holding meetings.

200. If the heart is not in the work, the benefits from the exercise are not the same.

Healthful Living, 129.

IF WORK is performed without the heart's being in it, it is simply drudgery, and the benefit which should result from the exercise is not gained.

201. Morning walking or gardening in the open air is the surest way to prevent respiratory and many other illnesses.

Healthful Living,130.

MORNING exercise, in walking in the free, invigorating air of heaven, or cultivating flowers, small fruits, and vegetables, is necessary to a healthful circulation of the blood. It is the surest safeguard against colds, coughs, congestions of the brain and lungs, inflammation of the liver, the kidneys, and the lungs, and a hundred other diseases.

202. Moderate walking after a meal benefits the digestion.

Healthful Living, 130.

EXERCISE will aid the work of digestion. To walk out after a meal, hold the head erect, put back the shoulders, and exercise moderately, will be a great benefit. The mind will be diverted from self to the beauties of nature. The less the attention is called to the stomach after a meal, the better.

203. Moderate exercise benefits digestion, but heavy physical or mental exercise immediately after a full meal hinders the digestion.

Testimonies, vol. 2, 413.

MY BROTHER, your brain is benumbed. A man who disposes of the quantity of food that you do should be a laboring man. Exercise is important to digestion and to a healthy condition of body and mind. You need physical exercise. You move and act as if you were wooden, as though you had no elasticity. Healthy, active exercise is what you need. This will invigorate the mind. Neither study nor violent exercise should be engaged in immediately after a full meal; this would be a violation of the laws of the system. Immediately after eating there is a strong draft upon the nervous energy. The brain force is called into active exercise to assist the stomach; therefore, when the mind or body is taxed heavily after eating, the process of digestion is hindered. The vitality of the system, which is needed to carry on the work in one direction, is called away and set to work in another.

204. The exercise needed to expand the lungs and strengthen the voice will prolong life.

Healthful Living, 133.

BY JUDICIOUS exercise they may expand the chest and strengthen the muscles. . . . By giving heed to proper instruction, by following health principles in regard to the expansion of the lungs and culture of the voice, our young men and women may become speakers that can be heard, and the exercise necessary to this accomplishment will prolong life.

205. Exercise in the open air and sunshine benefits mind and body, and is one of God's best gifts to man.

Christian Temperance and Bible Hygiene, 173.

PROPER exercise in the open air and genial sunshine, ranks among God's highest and richest blessings to man. It gives form and strength to the physical organism, and, all other habits being equal, is the surest safeguard against disease and premature decay. Being man's natural condition, it also gives buoyancy and strength to thought, and the mind maintains a healthful balance, free from the extremes resulting from artificial life.

206. Physical inaction, by lessening the mental and moral powers, hinders Heaven's communication with man.

Education, 209.

PHYSICAL inaction lessens not only mental but moral power. The brain nerves that connect with the whole system are the medium through which Heaven communicates with man and affects the inmost life. Whatever hinders the circulation of the electric current in the nervous system, thus weakening the vital powers and lessening mental susceptibility, makes it more difficult to arouse the moral nature.

207. Children need to spend the first eight to ten years of their life in the field or garden, laying the foundation for their physical development.

Education, 208.

CHILDREN should not be long confined within doors, nor should they be required to apply themselves closely to study until a good foundation has been laid for physical development. For the first eight or ten years of a child's life the field or garden is the best schoolroom, the mother the best teacher, nature the best lesson book. Even when the child is old enough to attend school, his health should be regarded as of greater importance than a knowledge of books. He should be surrounded with the conditions most favorable to both physical and mental growth.

208. The schoolroom should be combined with physical activity in order to enable the mental powers to function at their highest capacity.

Education, 207.

THE whole body is designed for action; and unless the physical powers are kept in health by active exercise, the mental powers cannot long be used to their highest capacity. The physical inaction which seems almost inevitable in the schoolroom together with other unhealthful conditions makes it a trying place for children, especially for those of feeble constitution.

209. Regular outdoor exercise, combined with the studies, will improve mental and physical strength, as well as prevent physical disease.

Education, 208.

THE child is not alone in the danger from want of air and exercise. In the higher as well as the lower schools these essentials to health are still too often neglected. Many a student sits day after day in a close room bending over his books, his chest so contracted that he cannot take a full, deep breath, his blood moving sluggishly, his feet cold, his head hot. The body not being sufficiently nourished, the muscles are weakened, and the whole system is enervated and diseased. Often such students become lifelong invalids. They might have come from school with increased physical as well as mental strength, had they pursued their studies under proper conditions, with regular exercise in the sunlight and the open air.

210. Students with limited time will find that physical exercise will make them more efficient in their studies.

Education, 208–209.

THE student who with limited time and means is struggling to gain an education should realize that time spent in physical exercise is not lost. He who continually pores over his books will find, after a time, that the mind has lost its freshness. Those who give proper attention to physical development will make greater advancement in literary lines than they would if their entire time were devoted to study.

211. Insufficient physical exercise, by leaving the brain congested, lessens self control and is, thus,

largely responsible for the present tide of corruption.

Education, 209.

AGAIN, excessive study, by increasing the flow of blood to the brain, creates morbid excitability that tends to lessen the power of self-control, and too often gives sway to impulse or caprice. Thus the door is opened to impurity. The misuse or nonuse of the physical powers is largely responsible for the tide of corruption that is overspreading the world. "Pride, fullness of bread, and abundance of idleness," are as deadly foes to human progress in this generation as when they led to the destruction of Sodom.

212. Teachers should teach their pupils that physical exercise is essential to right thinking and purity of thought.

Education, 209.

TEACHERS should understand these things, and should instruct their pupils in these lines. Teach the students that right living depends on right thinking, and that physical activity is essential to purity of thought.

213. Gymnastic exercises must have careful supervision.

Education, 210.

THE question of suitable recreation for their pupils is one that teachers often find perplexing. Gymnastic exercises fill a useful place in many schools; but without careful supervision they are often carried to excess. In the gymnasium many youth, by their attempted feats of strength, have done themselves lifelong injury.

214. Useful, outdoor labor, combined with the studies, is more beneficial than gymnastic exercises and makes them unnecessary.

Healthful Living, 28.

WHEN useful labor is combined with study, there is no need of gymnastic exercises; and much more benefit is derived from work performed in the open air than from indoor exercise, The farmer and the mechanic each have physical exercise; yet the farmer is much the healthier of the two, for nothing short of the invigorating air and sunshine will fully meet the wants of the system. The farmer finds in his labor all the movements that were ever practiced in the gymnasium. And his movement room is the open fields; the canopy of heaven is its roof, the solid earth is its floor.

215. When teachers turn from God's plan for exercise—useful, practical work—it is likened to the days of Noah.

Spalding and Magan, 70.

I WAS speaking to teachers in messages of reproof. All teachers need exercise, a change of employment. God has pointed out what this should be—useful, practical work; but you have turned away from God's plan to follow human inventions, and that to the detriment of the spiritual. Not a jot or a tittle of the after influence of an education in that line will fit you to meet the severe conflicts in the last days. What kind of education are our teachers and students receiving? Has God devised and planned this kind of exercise

for you, or is it brought in by human inventions and human imaginations? How is the mind prepared for contemplation and meditation, and serious thoughts, and the earnest, contrite prayer, coming from hearts subdued by the Holy Spirit of God; "As it was in the days of Noah, so shall it be when the Son of Man is revealed." "And God saw that the wickedness of man was great in the earth, and that every imagination of the thoughts of his heart was only evil continually."

216. The best conducted exercise in a gymnasium cannot compare to the benefits of recreation in the open air; and sports in general have a disturbing influence.

Education, 210.

EXERCISE in a gymnasium, however well conducted, cannot supply the place of recreation in the open air, and for this our schools should afford better opportunity. Vigorous exercise the pupils must have. Few evils are more to be dreaded than indolence and aimlessness. Yet the tendency of most athletic sports is a subject of anxious thought to those who have at heart the well-being of the youth. Teachers are troubled as they consider the influence of these sports both on the student's progress in school and on his success in afterlife. The games that occupy so much of his time are diverting the mind from study. They are not helping to prepare the youth for practical, earnest work in life. Their influence does not tend toward refinement, generosity, or real manliness.

217. Games of football are likened to the experience of Israel at mount Sinai, when they rose up to play.

Spalding and Magan, 69.

BUT what returns have our young people made to the Lord? Has it been as it was with the people of Israel on that most solemn occasion described in Exodus? Moses had gone up into the Mount to receive instruction from the Lord, and the whole congregation should have been in humble attitude before God; but instead of that, they ate and drank and rose up to play. Has there been a similar experience in Battle Creek? Have not many lost their hold on God? Did the exercise in games of football bring the participants into more close relation to God?

218. The intensely absorbing sports are Satan's snares to have us labeled in heaven as "lovers of pleasure more than lovers of God."

Spalding and Magan, 69–70.

IN THE night seasons messages have been given to me to give to you in Battle Creek, and to all our schools. While it is in the order of God that physical powers shall be trained as well as the mental, yet the physical exercises should in character be in complete harmony with the lessons given to the world and should be seen in the lives of Christians, so that in education and self-training the heavenly intelligences should not record in the books that students and the teachers in our schools are "Lovers of pleasure more than lovers of God." This is the record now being made of a large number, "Lovers of pleasure more than lovers of God." Thus

Satan and his angels are laying their snares for your souls, and he is working in a certain way upon teachers and pupils to induce them to engage in certain exercises and amusements which become intensely absorbing, but which are of a character to strengthen the lower powers, and create appetites and passions that will take the lead and counteract most decidedly the operations and working of the Holy Spirit of God upon the human heart.

219. Teachers are not in the work of God to invent games that bring the sacred down to the level of the common.

Spalding and Magan, 70.

WHAT saith the Holy Spirit to you? What was its power and influence upon your hearts during the General Conference and the conference in other states? Have you taken special heed to yourself? Have the teachers in the school felt that they must take heed: If God has appointed them as educators of the youth, they are also "overseers of the flock." They are not in the school work to invent plans for exercises and games to educate pupils; not there to bring down sacred things on a level with the common.

220. Many invalids will never improve until they rise above their aches and fears and engage in useful labor.

Testimonies, vol. 3, 76.

THOUSANDS are sick and dying around us who might get well and live if they would; but their imagination holds them. They fear that they will be made worse if they labor or exercise, when this is just the change they need to make them well. Without this they never can improve. They should exercise the power of the will, rise above their aches and debility, engage in useful employment, and forget that they have aching backs, sides, lungs, and heads. Neglecting to exercise the entire body, or a portion of it, will bring on morbid conditions. Inaction of any of the organs of the body will be followed by a decrease in size and strength of the muscles, and will cause the blood to flow sluggishly through the blood vessels.

If there are duties to be done in your domestic life, you do not think it possible that you could do them, but you depend upon others. Sometimes it is exceedingly inconvenient for you to obtain the help you need. You frequently expend double the strength required to perform the task, in planning and searching for someone to do the work for you. If you would only bring your mind to do these little acts and family duties yourself, you would be blessed and strengthened in it, and your influence in the cause of God would be far greater.

221. The best of health cannot be had without the best of circulation, and this is impossible without exercise in the open air.

Testimonies, vol. 2, 525.

THE chief if not the only reason why many become invalids is that the blood does not circulate freely, and the changes in the vital fluid, which are necessary to life and health, do not take place. They have not given their bodies exercise nor their lungs food, which is pure, fresh air; therefore it is impossible for the blood to be vitalized, and it pursues its course sluggishly through the system. The more we exercise, the better will be the circulation of the blood. More people die for want of exercise than through overfatigue; very many more rust out than wear out. Those who accustom themselves to proper exercise in the open air will generally have a good and vigorous circulation. We are more dependent upon the air we breathe than upon the food we eat. Men and women, young and old, who desire health, and who would enjoy active life, should remember that they cannot have these without a good circulation. Whatever their business and inclinations, they should make up their minds to exercise in the open air as much as they can. They should feel it a religious duty to overcome the conditions of health which have kept them confined indoors, deprived of exercise in the open air.

222. Invalids, if at all possible, must exercise to regain their warmth, as well as their health.

Testimonies, vol. 2, 526.

SOME invalids become willful in the matter and refuse to be convinced of the great importance of daily outdoor exercise, whereby they may obtain a supply of pure air. For fear of taking cold, they persist, from year to year, in having their own way and living in an atmosphere almost destitute of vitality. It is impossible for this class to have a healthy circulation. The entire system suffers for want of exercise and pure air. The skin becomes debilitated and more sensitive to any change in the atmosphere. Additional clothing is put on, and the heat of the room increased. The next day they require a little more heat and a little more clothing in order to feel perfectly warm, and thus they humor every changing feeling until they have but little vitality to endure any cold. Some may inquire: "What shall we do? Would you have us remain cold?" If you add clothing, let it be but little, and exercise, if possible, to regain the heat you need. If you positively cannot engage in active exercise, warm yourselves by the fire; but as soon as you are warm, lay off your extra clothing and remove from the fire. If those who can, would engage in some active employment to take the mind from themselves, they would generally forget that they were chilly and would not receive harm. You should lower the temperature of your room as soon as you have regained your natural warmth. For invalids who have feeble lungs, nothing can be worse than an overheated atmosphere.

223. Brisk, outdoor exercise improves the circulation of the congested organs by drawing the blood to the surface, and this will restore the health to many invalids.

Testimonies, vol. 2, 530.

MANY labor under the mistaken idea that if they have taken cold, they must carefully exclude the outside air and increase the temperature of their room until it is excessively hot. The system may be deranged, the pores closed by waste matter, and the internal organs suffering more or less inflammation, because the blood has been chilled back from the surface and thrown upon them. At this time, of all others, the lungs should not be deprived of pure, fresh air. If pure air is ever necessary, it is when any part of the system, as the lungs or stomach, is diseased. Judicious exercise would induce the blood to the surface, and thus relieve the internal organs. Brisk, yet not violent exercise in the open air, with cheerfulness of spirits, will promote the circulation, giving healthful glow to the skin, and sending the blood, vitalized by the pure air, to the extremities. The diseased stomach will find relief by exercise. Physicians frequently advise invalids to visit foreign countries, to go to the springs, or to ride upon the ocean, in order to regain health; when, in nine cases out of ten, if they would eat temperately and engage in healthful exercise with a cheerful spirit, they would regain health and save time and money. Exercise, and a free abundant use of the air and sunlight, blessings which Heaven has freely bestowed upon all would give life and strength to the emaciated invalid.

224. The tiredness and soreness after exercise of previously underused muscles is evidence of their awakening to life.

Testimonies, vol. 3, 78.

THOSE who are feeble and indolent should not yield to their inclination to be inactive, thus depriving themselves of air and sunlight, but should practice exercising out of doors in walking or working in the garden. They will become very much fatigued, but this will not injure them. You, my sister, will experience weariness, yet it will not hurt you; your rest will be sweeter after it. Inaction weakens the organs that are not exercised. And when these organs are used, pain and weariness are experienced, because the muscles have become feeble. It is not good policy to give up the use of certain muscles because pain is felt when they are exercised. The pain is frequently caused by the effort of nature to give life and vigor to those parts that have become partially lifeless through inaction. The motion of these long-disused muscles will cause pain, because nature is awakening them to life.

225. Invalids, take your thoughts off of yourself, give a trial to useful exercise and be convinced of its blessings.

Testimonies, vol. 2, 534.

INVALIDS, I advise you to venture something. Arouse your will power, and at least make a trial of this matter. Withdraw your thoughts and affections from yourselves. Walk out by faith. Are you inclined to center your thoughts upon yourselves, fearing to exercise, and fearing that if you expose yourself to the air you will lose your life; resist these thoughts and feelings. Do not yield to your diseased imagination. If you fail in the trial, you can but die. And what if you do die? One life might better be lost than many sacrificed. The whims and notions which you cherish are not only destroying your own life, but injuring those whose lives are more valuable than yours. But the course we recommend will not deprive you of life or injure you. You will derive benefit from it. You need not be rash or reckless; commence moderately at first to have more air and exercise, and continue your reform until you become useful, a blessing to your families and to all around you. Let your judgment be convinced that exercise, sunlight, and air are the blessings which Heaven has provided to make the sick well and to keep in health those who are not sick. God does not deprive you of these free, Heaven-bestowed blessings, but you have punished yourselves by closing your doors against them. Properly used, these simple yet powerful agents will assist nature to overcome real difficulties, if such exist, and will give healthy tone to the mind and vigor to the body.

The True Remedies—VI
Proper Diet

226. Proper diet is a moral issue.

Christian Temperance and Bible Hygiene, 76.

THE diet affects both physical and moral health. How carefully, then, should mothers study to supply the table with the most simple, healthful food, in order that the digestive organs may not be weakened, the nerves unbalanced, or the instruction which they give their children counteracted.

227. Diet affects the quality and efficiency of our usefulness in life.

Healthful Living, 78.

IS MY diet such as will bring me in a position where I can accomplish the greatest amount of good?

228. God's chosen diet for us of grains, fruits, nuts, and vegetables is the most healthful.

Counsels on Diet and Foods, 81.

GRAINS, fruits, nuts and vegetables constitute the diet chosen for us by our Creator. These foods, prepared in as simple and natural a manner as possible, are the most healthful and nourishing. They impart a strength, a power of endurance, and a vigor of intellect, that are not afforded by a more complex and stimulating diet.

229. Milk and cream may also be part of the most healthful diet.

Healthful Living, 78.

FRUITS, grains, and vegetables, prepared in a simple way, free from spice and grease of all kinds, make, with milk and cream, the most healthful diet. They impart nourishment to the body, and give a power of endurance and vigor of intellect that are not produced by a stimulating diet.

230. Providentially, each country has adequate types of food for proper nutrition.

Counsels on Diet and Foods, 94.

IN THE providence of God, every country produces articles of food containing the nourishment necessary for the upbuilding of the system.

231. The most wholesome articles of food vary from individual to individual.

Healthful Living, 78.

PEOPLE cannot all eat the same things. Some articles of food that are wholesome and palatable to one person may be hurtful to another. So it is impossible to make an unvarying rule by which to regulate every one's dietetic habits.

232. The stomach should have periods of rest between meals.

Healthful Living, 84.

A SECOND meal should never be eaten until the stomach has had time to rest from the labor of digesting the preceding meal.

233. There should be at least five hours between meals.

Healthful Living, 82.

THE stomach must have careful attention. . . . After it has done its work for one meal, do not crowd more work upon it before it has had a chance to rest, and before a sufficient supply of gastric juice is provided. Five hours at least should be given between each meal, and always bear in mind that if you would give it a trial, you would find two meals better than three.

234. Two meals a day is best for most people, but if necessary a very light third meal may be taken.

Healthful Living, 84.

MOST people enjoy better health while eating two meals a day than three; others, under their existing circumstances, may require something to eat at supper time; but this meal should be very light. Let no one think himself a criterion for all, that every one must do exactly as he does.

235. Children on two meals a day are generally in better physical, social, and spiritual health.

The Health Reformer, May 1, 1877.

FOR more than twelve years we have taken only two meals each day, of plain, unstimulating food. During that time, we have had almost constantly the care of children, varying in age from three to thirteen years. We worked gradually and carefully to change their habit of eating three times a day to two; we also worked cautiously to change their diet from stimulating food, as meat, rich gravies, pies, cakes, butter, spices, etc., to simple, wholesome fruits, vegetables, and grains. The consequence has been that our children have not been troubled with the various maladies to which children are more or less subject. They occasionally take cold by reason of carelessness, but this seldom makes them sick.

We have, as an occasional experiment, changed the number of their daily meals from two to three; but the result was not good. In the morning their breath was offensive; and after testing the matter for a few weeks, we were thoroughly convinced that the children were better upon two meals a day than upon three; and we therefore returned to our former system, with marked improvement in the health of the children as a result. If tempted with the sight of food prepared for others, they incline to think they are hungry, but usually they do not miss or think about the third meal. Children reared in this way are much more easily controlled than those who are indulged in eating everything their appetite craves, and at all times. They are usually cheerful, contented, and healthy. Even the most stubborn, passionate, and wayward, have become submissive, patient, and possessed of self-control by persistently following up this order of diet, united with a firm but kind management in regard to other matters.

236. Children as young as one to three years of age can do well on two meals a day.

Review and Herald, April 14, 1868.

THE term properly called infancy, requires several changes as to the periods of taking food. Before birth it is receiving nourishment constantly. And the changes from this to the establishment of only two meals a day, which may, in most children, be done from the ages of one to three years, must be gradual.

237. The third meal should never be a hearty one, and most would be healthier to skip it entirely.

Healthful Living, 82.

IT IS quite a common custom with the people of the world to eat three times a day, besides eating at irregular intervals between meals; and the last meal is generally the most hearty, and is often taken just before retiring. This is reversing the natural order; a hearty meal should never be taken so late in the day. Should these persons change their practice, and eat but two meals a day, and nothing between meals, not even an apple, a nut, or any kind of fruit, the result would be seen in a good appetite and greatly improved health.

238. Mealtime is to be a pleasant and grateful time.

Healthful Living, 85.

AT MEAL time cast off care and taxing thought. Do not be hurried, but eat slowly and with cheerfulness, your heart filled with gratitude to God for all his blessings.

239. Choose wisely, ask the Lord's blessing, and then do not worry about the effects of your food.

Healthful Living, 85.

SOME health reformers are constantly worrying for fear their food, however simple and healthful, will hurt them. To these let me say, Do not think that your food is going to hurt you; but when you have eaten according to your best judgment, and have asked the Lord to bless the food, believe that he has heard your prayer, and be at rest.

240. For physical and spiritual health, eat slowly, and, if your time is limited, eat less.

Healthful Living, 86.

IN ORDER to have healthy digestion, food should be eaten slowly. Those who wish to avoid dyspepsia, and those who realize the obligation to keep all their powers in a condition which will enable them to render the best service to God, will do well to remember this. If your time to eat is limited, do not bolt your food, but eat less, and eat slowly.

241. Slow eating improves the gratification of the taste, and by increased mixing with the saliva it improves the nutrition received.

Healthful Living, 86.

EAT slowly, and allow the saliva to mingle with the food. The more liquid there is taken into the stomach with the meals, the more difficult it is for the food to digest. . . . The benefit you derive from your food does not depend so much on the quantity eaten, as on its thorough digestion, nor the gratification of the taste so much on the amount of food swallowed as on the length of time it remains in the mouth.

242. Fluids with meals decrease the saliva, and, if cold, they arrest the digestion until warmed by the stomach.

Healthful Living, 89.

TAKEN with meals, water diminishes the flow of the salivary glands; and the colder the water the greater the injury to the stomach. Ice water or iced lemonade, drunk with meals, will arrest digestion until the system has imparted sufficient warmth to the stomach to enable it to take up its work again.

243. Pure water is the only necessary beverage; but if it, or any other fluid, is drunk with meals, it must be absorbed before digestion can be completed.

Healthful Living, 89.

FOOD should not be washed down; no drink is needed with meals. Eat slowly, and allow the saliva to mingle with the food. The more liquid there is taken into the stomach with the meals, the more difficult it is for the food to digest; for the liquid must be first absorbed. . . . Hot drinks are debilitating; and besides, those who indulge in their use become slaves to the habit. . . . Do not eat largely of salt; give up bottled pickles; keep fiery spiced food out of your stomach; eat fruit with your meals, and the irritation which calls for so much drink will cease to exist. But if anything is needed to quench thirst, pure water, drunk some little time before or after a meal, is all that nature requires. . . . Water is the best liquid possible to cleanse the tissues.

244. It is advisable to take something warm into the stomach for breakfast, because cold foods require digestive vitality to bring them to body temperature.

Testimonies, vol. 2, 603.

I WOULD advise all to take something warm into the stomach every morning at least. You can do this without much labor. You can make graham gruel. If the graham flour is too coarse, sift it, and while the gruel is hot, add milk. This will make a most palatable and healthful dish for the campground. And if your bread is dry, crumb it into the gruel, and it will be enjoyed. I do not approve of eating much cold food, for the reason that the vitality must be drawn from the system to warm the food until it becomes of the same temperature as the stomach before the work of digestion can be carried on. Another very simple yet wholesome dish is beans boiled or baked. Dilute a portion of them with water, add milk or cream, and make a broth; the bread can be used as in graham gruel.

245. Nervous brain energy is required to throw off the effects of decaying excess food that is eaten.

Healthful Living, 87.

IF MORE food is eaten than can be digested and appropriated, a decaying mass accumulates in the stomach, causing an offensive breath, and a bad taste in the mouth. The vital powers are exhausted in an effort to throw off the excess, and the brain is robbed of nerve force.

246. There is great benefit in a nourishing, well-regulated diet prepared with the family and not just visitors in mind.

Testimonies, vol. 2, 485.

ONE family in particular have needed all the benefits they could receive from the reform in diet, yet these very ones have been completely backslidden. Meat and butter have been used by them quite freely, and spices have not been entirely discarded. This family could have received great benefit from a nourishing, well-regulated diet. The head of the family needed plain, nutritious food. His habits were sedentary, and his blood moved sluggishly through the system. He could not, like others, have the benefit of healthful exercise; therefore his food should have been of the right quality and quantity. There has not been in this family the right management in regard to diet; there has been irregularity. There should have been a specified time for each meal, and the food should have been prepared in a simple form and free from grease but pains should have been taken to have it nutritious, healthful, and inviting. In this family, as also in many others, a special parade has been made for visitors, many dishes prepared and frequently made too rich, so that those seated at the table would be tempted to eat to excess. Then in the absence of company there was a great reaction, a falling off in the preparations brought on the table. The diet was spare and lacked nourishment. It was considered not so much matter "just for ourselves." The meals were frequently picked up, and the regular time for eating not regarded. Every member of the family was injured by such management. It is a sin for any of our sisters to make such great preparations for visitors, and wrong their own families by a spare diet which will fail to nourish the system.

247. Excess eating of even good food is gluttony, weakening the energies of the soul.

Testimonies, vol. 2, 412.

MY BROTHER, you are far from God; you are in a state of backsliding. You do not possess noble moral courage. You yield to your own desires instead of denying self. In seeking after happiness, you have attended places of amusement which God does not approve, and in so doing have weakened your own soul. My brother, you have much to learn. You indulge your appetite by eating more food than your system can convert into good blood. It is sin to be intemperate in the quantity of food eaten, even if the quality is unobjectionable. Many feel that, if they do not eat meat and the grosser articles of food, they may eat of simple food until they cannot well eat more. This is a mistake. Many professed health reformers are nothing less than gluttons. They lay upon the digestive organs so great a burden that the vitality of the system is exhausted in the effort to dispose of

it. It also has a depressing influence upon the intellect, for the brain nerve power is called upon to assist the stomach in its work. Overeating, even of the simplest food, benumbs the sensitive nerves of the brain and weakens its vitality. Overeating has a worse effect upon the system than over working; the energies of the soul are more effectually prostrated by intemperate eating than by intemperate working.

248. Excess food may cause obesity, or it may cause thinness.

The Ministry of Healing, 240.

SOME grow corpulent because the system is clogged; others become thin and feeble because their vital powers are exhausted in disposing of an excess of food.

249. The system is clogged by excess food and extracts fewer nutrients than when less food is eaten.

Testimonies, vol. 2, 412.

THE digestive organs should never be burdened with a quantity or quality of food which it will tax the system to appropriate. All that is taken into the stomach above what the system can use to convert into good blood, clogs the machinery; for it cannot be made into either flesh or blood, and its presence burdens the liver and produces a morbid condition of the system. The stomach is overworked in its efforts to dispose of it, and then there is a sense of languor, which is interpreted to mean hunger; and without allowing the digestive organs time to rest from their severe labor, to recruit their energies another immoderate amount is taken into the stomach, to set the weary machinery again in motion. The system receives less nourishment from too great a quantity of food, even of the right quality, than from a moderate quantity taken at regular periods.

250. Exercise helps counteract some of the effects of excess eating.

Testimonies, vol. 3, 489.

MINISTERS, teachers, and students do not become as intelligent as they should in regard to the necessity of physical exercise in the open air. They neglect this duty, which is most essential for the preservation of health. They closely apply their minds to books and eat the allowance of a laboring man. Under such habits some grow corpulent, because the system is clogged. Others become lean, feeble, and weak because their vital powers are exhausted in throwing off the excess of food; the liver becomes burdened and unable to throw off the impurities in the blood, and sickness is the result. If physical exercise were combined with mental exertion, the blood would be quickened in its circulation, the action of the heart would be more perfect, impure matter would be thrown off, and new life and vigor would be experienced in every part of the body.

251. Excessively hot foods tend to debilitate the stomach.

Healthful Living, 91.

VERY hot food ought not to be taken into the stomach. Soups, puddings, and other articles of the kind, are often eaten too hot, and as a consequence the stomach is debilitated. Let them become partly cooled before they are eaten.

252. Ripe but undecayed fruit is from the Lord.

Healthful Living, 79.

GOOD, ripe, undecayed fruit is a thing for which we should thank the Lord, for it is beneficial to health.

253. Hot or new, raised bread is difficult to digest.

The Ministry of Healing, 301.

WHEN hot or new, raised bread of any kind is difficult of digestion. It should never appear on the table. This rule does not, however, apply to unleavened bread.

254. Bread should be well done and never sour, heavy, or made with milk.

Healthful Living, 80.

BREAD should never have the slightest taint of sourness. It should be cooked until it is most thoroughly done. Thus all softness and stickiness will be avoided. . . . Milk should not be used in place of water in bread making. All this is extra expense, and is not wholesome. If the bread thus made is allowed to stand over in warm weather, and is then broken open, there will frequently be seen long strings like cobwebs. Such bread soon causes fermentation to take place in the stomach. . . . Every housekeeper should feel it her duty to educate herself to make good sweet bread in the most inexpensive manner, and the family should refuse to have upon the table bread that is heavy and sour, for it is injurious.

255. Hot baking-powder biscuits should never be eaten.

Healthful Living, 81.

HOT biscuit raised with soda or baking-powder should never appear upon our tables. Such compounds are unfit to enter the stomach.

256. Hot soda biscuits with butter are an abuse to the digestive organs.

Healthful Living, 95.

HOT soda biscuits are often spread with butter, and eaten as a choice diet; but the feeble digestive organs cannot but feel the abuse placed upon them.

257. A disturbance is created when a great variety of food is eaten at one meal.

Healthful Living, 82.

IT IS not well to take a great variety of food at one meal. When a variety of foods that do not agree are crowded into the stomach at one meal, what can we expect but that a disturbance will be created?

258. Have one meal of bread and fruit, and one of vegetables, and avoid the combination of eggs, milk, and sugar.

Healthful Living, 82.

I ADVISE the people to give up sweet puddings or custards made with eggs and milk and sugar, and to eat the best home-made bread, both graham and white, with dried or green fruits, and let that be the only course for one meal; then let the next meal be of nicely prepared vegetables.

259. For the best health, avoid eating vegetables and fruit at the same meal, especially if the stomach is feeble.

Healthful Living, 82.

IF WE would preserve the best health, we should avoid eating vegetables and fruit at the same meal. If the stomach is feeble, there will be distress, and the brain will be confused, and unable to put forth mental effort. Have fruit at one meal and vegetables at the next.

260. When the mother serves improper foods, it is more difficult to arouse the moral sensibilities of the children, and impossible for them to perfect Christian character.

Christian Temperance and Bible Hygiene, 46.

IT IS impossible for those who give the reins to appetite to attain to Christian perfection. The moral sensibilities of your children cannot be easily aroused, unless you are careful in the selection of their food. Many a mother sets a table that is a snare to her family. Fleshmeats, butter, cheese, rich pastry, spiced foods, and condiments are freely partaken of by both old and young. These things do their work in deranging the stomach, exciting the nerves, and enfeebling the intellect. The blood making organs cannot convert such things into good blood. The grease cooked in the food renders it difficult of digestion. The effect of cheese is deleterious. Fine-flour bread does not impart to the system the nourishment that is to be found in unbolted wheat bread. Its common use will not keep the system in the best condition. Spices at first irritate the tender coating of the stomach, but finally destroy the natural sensitiveness of this delicate membrane. The blood becomes fevered, the animal propensities are aroused, while the moral and intellectual powers are weakened, and become servants to the baser passions. The mother should study to set a simple yet nutritious diet before her family.

261. Condiments and spices cause a temporary stimulus of digestion followed by depression.

Healthful Living, 92.

CONDIMENTS and spices, used in the preparation of food for the table, aid digestion in the same way that tea, coffee, and liquor are supposed to help the laboring man to perform his task. After the immediate effects are gone, those who use them drop as far below par as they were elevated above par by these stimulating substances. The system is weakened, the blood contaminated, and inflammation is the sure result. The less frequently condiments and desserts are placed on our tables, the better it will be for all who partake of the food.

262. Flesh meats, rich foods, and an impoverished diet all form a poor quality of blood.

Testimonies, vol. 2, 368.

FLESH meats will depreciate the blood. Cook meat with spices, and eat it with rich cakes and pies, and you have a bad quality of blood. The system is too heavily taxed in disposing of this kind of food. The mince pies and the pickles, which should never find a place in any human stomach, will give a miserable quality of blood. And a poor quality of food, cooked in an improper manner, and insufficient in quantity, cannot make good blood. Flesh meats and rich food, and an impoverished diet, will produce the same results.

263. Large quantities of milk and sugar eaten together are injurious.

Testimonies, vol. 2, 368.

NOW in regard to milk and sugar: I know of persons who have become frightened at the health reform, and said they would have nothing to do with it, because it has spoken against a free use of these things. Changes should be made with great care, and we should move cautiously and wisely. We want to take that course which will recommend itself to the intelligent men and women of the land. Large quantities of milk and sugar eaten together are injurious. They impart impurities to the system. Animals from which milk is obtained are not always healthy. They may be diseased. A cow may be apparently well in the morning, and die before night. Then she was diseased in the morning, and her milk was diseased; but you did not know it. The animal creation is diseased. Flesh meats are diseased. Could we know that animals were in perfect health, I would recommend that people eat flesh meats sooner than large quantities of milk and sugar. It would not do the injury that milk and sugar do. Sugar clogs the system. It hinders the working of the living machine.

264. Part of the corruption of the antediluvian world was caused by the eating of flesh meats.

Christian Temperance and Bible Hygiene, 43.

SINCE the first surrender to appetite, mankind have been growing more and more self indulgent, until health has been sacrificed on the altar of appetite. The inhabitants of the antediluvian world were intemperate in eating and drinking. They would have flesh meats, although God had at that time given man no permission to eat animal food. They ate and drank till the indulgence of their depraved appetite knew no bounds, and they became so corrupt that God could bear with them no longer. Their cup of iniquity was full, and he cleansed the earth of its moral pollution by a flood.

265. Esau permanently traded his birthright for the indulgence of one coveted dish.

Christian Temperance and Bible Hygiene, 43.

ESAU had a strong desire for a particular article of food, and he had so long gratified himself that he did not feel the necessity of turning from the tempting, coveted dish. He allowed his imagination to dwell upon it until the power of appetite bore down every other consideration, and controlled him. He thought he would suffer great inconvenience, and even death, if he could not have that particular dish. The more he reflected upon it, the more his desire strengthened, until his birthright lost its value and sacredness in his sight,

and he bartered it away. He flattered himself that he could dispose of his birthright at will, and buy it back at pleasure; but when he sought to regain it, even at a great sacrifice, he was not able to do so. He then bitterly repented of his rashness, his folly, his madness; but it was all in vain. He had despised the blessing, and the Lord had removed it from him forever.

266. Reason has abdicated to the indulgence of appetite, resulting in increased crime and disease.

Christian Temperance and Bible Hygiene, 44.

CRIME and disease have increased with every succeeding generation. Intemperance in eating and drinking, and the indulgence of the baser passions, have benumbed the nobler faculties of man. Reason, instead of being the ruler, has come to be the slave of appetite to an alarming extent. An increasing desire for rich food has been indulged, until it has become the fashion to crowd all the delicacies possible into the stomach. Especially at parties of pleasure is the appetite indulged with but little restraint. Rich dinners and late suppers are served, consisting of highly seasoned meats, with rich sauces, cakes, pies, ices, tea, coffee, etc. No wonder that, with such a diet, people have sallow complexions, and suffer untold agonies from dyspepsia.

267. God has said that we are to eat neither the blood nor the fat of animals.

Leviticus 3:17.

IT SHALL be a perpetual statute for your generations throughout all your dwellings, that ye eat neither fat nor blood.

268. Many diseases are caused by poor quality blood, resulting from eating animal fat and blood.

Healthful Living, 93.

MEAT is served reeking with fat, because it suits the perverted taste. Both the blood and the fat of animals is consumed as a luxury. But the Lord has given special directions that these should not be eaten. Why? Because their use would make a diseased current of blood in the human system. Disregard of the Lord's special directions has brought many diseases upon human beings.

269. Because of persistent rebellion, God permitted the people after the flood to eat animal food, which rapidly decreased their stature and longevity.

Counsels on Diet and Foods, 373.

AFTER the flood the people ate largely of animal food. God saw that the ways of man were corrupt, and that he was disposed to exalt himself proudly against his Creator and to follow the inclinations of his own heart. And He permitted that long-lived race to eat animal food to shorten their sinful lives. Soon after the flood the race began to rapidly decrease in size, and in length of years.

270. In these last days meat-eating is related to mental and moral degeneracy, as well as to physical degeneracy.

Healthful Living, 98.

SPEAKING in support of this diet, they said that without it they were weak in physical strength. But the words of our Teacher to us were, "As a man thinketh, so is he." The flesh of dead animals was not the original food for man. Man was permitted to eat it after the flood, because all vegetation had been destroyed. . . . Since the flood the human race has been shortening the period of its existence. Physical, mental, and moral degeneracy is rapidly increasing in these last days.

271. Meat-eating strengthens the animal passions while weakening the intellectual and moral powers, and it should be replaced by a nourishing diet.

Testimonies, vol. 2, 63.

AFTER they have reduced their physical strength by a reduced quantity and a poor quality of food, some conclude that their former way of living is the best. The system must be nourished. Yet we do not hesitate to say that flesh meat is not necessary of health or strength. If used it is because a depraved appetite craves it. Its use excites the animal propensities to increased activity and strengthens the animal passions. When the animal propensities are increased, the intellectual and moral powers are decreased. The use of the flesh of animals tends to cause a grossness of body and benumbs the fine sensibilities of the mind.

272. The fluids and flesh of the animal become the fluids and flesh of the consumer, increasing the likelihood of contracting disease tenfold.

Testimonies, vol. 2, 63.

WILL the people who are preparing to become holy, pure, and refined, that they may be introduced into the society of heavenly angels, continue to take the life of God's creatures and subsist on their flesh and enjoy it as a luxury? From what the Lord has shown me, this order of things will be changed, and God's peculiar people will exercise temperance in all things. Those who subsist largely upon flesh cannot avoid eating the meat of animals which are to a greater or less degree diseased. The process of fitting animals for market produces in them disease; and fitted in as healthful manner as they can be, they become heated and diseased by driving before they reach the market. The fluids and flesh of these diseased animals are received directly into the blood, and pass into the circulation of the human body, becoming fluids and flesh of the same. These humors are introduced into the system. And if the person already has impure blood, it is greatly aggravated by the eating of the flesh of these animals. The liability to take disease is increased tenfold by meat-eating. The intellectual, the moral, and the physical powers are depreciated by the habitual use of flesh meats. Meat-eating deranges the system, beclouds the intellect, and blunts the moral sensibilities. We say to you, dear brother and sister, your safest course is to let meat alone.

273. God took flesh meats from the diet of the children of Israel in order that they could bear the divine credentials in their physical appearance.

Healthful Living, 96.

THE Lord intends to bring His people back to live upon simple fruits, vegetables, and grains. He led the children of Israel into the wilderness where they could not get a flesh diet; and He gave them the bread of heaven. "Man did eat angels' food." But they craved the flesh-pots of Egypt, and mourned and cried for flesh, notwithstanding the promise of the Lord that if they would submit to His will, He would carry them into the land of Canaan, and establish them there, a pure, holy, happy people, and that there should not be a feeble one in all their tribes; for He would take away all sickness from among them. . . . The Lord would have given them flesh had it been essential for their health, but He who had created and redeemed them led them through that long journey in the wilderness to educate, discipline, and train them in correct habits. The Lord understood what influence flesh eating has upon the human system. He would have a people that would, in their physical appearance, bear the divine credentials, notwithstanding their long journey.

274. God never designed that we get our vegetables and grains second-hand by the eating of other animals.

Healthful Living, 97.

THE diet of animals is vegetables and grains. Must the vegetables be animalized, must they be incorporated into the system of an animal, before we get them? Must we obtain our vegetable diet by eating the flesh of dead creatures? God provided food in its natural state for our first parents. He gave Adam charge of the garden, to dress it and to care for it, saying, To you it shall be for meat. One animal was not to destroy another animal for food.

275. It is a great error to believe that muscular strength is dependent upon meat-eating.

Healthful Living, 98.

ONE of the great errors that many insist upon is that muscular strength is dependent upon animal food. But the simple grains, fruits of the trees, and vegetables have all the nutritive properties necessary to make good blood. This a flesh diet cannot do.

276. The weakness first noted after leaving off meat is the natural depressant effect after leaving off a stimulant.

Healthful Living, 98–99.

THE weakness experienced on leaving off meat is one of the strongest arguments that I could present as a reason why you should discontinue its use. Those who eat meat feel stimulated after eating this food, and they suppose that they are made stronger. After they discontinue the use of meat, they may for a time feel weak, but when the system is cleansed from the effect of this diet, they no longer feel the weakness, and will cease to wish for that for which they have pleaded as essential to strength.

277. Meat is diseased, and even milk may not be safe.

Healthful Living, 79.

MEAT-EATING is doing its work, for the meat is diseased. We may not long be able to use even milk.

278. The eating of dead animals is the main cause of inflammatory diseases, tumors, and cancer.

Counsels on Diet and Foods, 388.

CANCERS, tumors, and all inflammatory diseases are largely caused by meat-eating. From the light God has given me, the prevalence of cancer and tumors is largely due to gross living on dead flesh.

279. When leaving off meat and rich foods, it may require some fasting and time for the appetite to relish the simple, but more nutritious diet.

Healthful Living, 93.

PERSONS who have indulged their appetite to eat freely of meat, highly seasoned gravies, and various kinds of rich cakes and preserves, cannot immediately relish a plain, wholesome, nutritious diet. Their taste is so perverted they have no appetite for a wholesome diet of fruits, plain bread, and vegetables. They need not expect to relish at first food so different from that in which they have been indulging. If they cannot at first enjoy plain food, they should fast until they can. That fast will prove to them of greater benefit than medicine, for the abused stomach will find the rest which it has long needed, and real hunger can be satisfied with a plain diet. It will take time for the taste to recover from the abuses it has received, and to gain its natural tone. But perseverance in a self-denying course of eating and drinking will soon make plain, wholesome food palatable, and it will be eaten with greater satisfaction than the epicure enjoys over his rich dainties.

280. When leaving off meat, be painstaking to have a nutritious and appetizing diet.

Testimonies, vol. 2, 63.

WE ADVISE you to change your habits of living; but while you do this we caution you to move understandingly. I am acquainted with families who have changed from a meat diet to one that is impoverished. Their food is so poorly prepared that the stomach loathes it; and such have told me that the health reform did not agree with them, that they were decreasing in physical strength. Here is one reason why some have not been successful in their efforts to simplify their food. They have a poverty-stricken diet. Food is prepared without painstaking, and there is a continual sameness. There should not be many kinds at any one meal, but all meals should not be composed of the same kinds of food without variation. Food should be prepared with simplicity, yet with a nicety which will invite the appetite. You should keep grease out of your food. It defiles any preparation of food you may make. Eat largely of fruits and vegetables.

281. The oil in the olives is preferred over butter.

Counsels on Health, 477.

OLIVES may be so prepared as to be eaten with good results at every meal. The advantages sought by the use of butter may be obtained by the eating of properly prepared olives. The oil in the olives relieves constipation, and for consumptives, and for those who have inflamed, irritated stomachs, it is better than any drug. As food it is better than any oil coming secondhand from animals.

282. We are to eat in strict accordance with the laws of health, avoiding not only harmful substances, but also an impoverished or unappetizing diet.

Testimonies, vol. 2, 367.

BUT what about an impoverished diet? I have spoken of the importance of the quantity and quality of food being in strict accordance with the laws of health. But we would not recommend an impoverished diet. I have been shown that many take a wrong view of the health reform and adopt too poor a diet. They subsist upon a cheap, poor quality of food, prepared without care or reference to the nourishment of the system. It is important that the food should by prepared with care, that the appetite, when not perverted, can relish it. Because we from principle discard the use of meat, butter, mince pies, spices, lard, and that which irritates the stomach and destroys health, the idea should never be given that it is of but little consequence what we eat.

283. It is a sacred work for mothers to teach their daughters how to prepare nutritious meals with nicety.

Testimonies, vol. 2, 538.

POOR cookery is slowly wearing away the life energies of thousands. It is dangerous to health and life to eat at some tables the heavy, sour bread and the other food prepared in keeping with it. Mothers, instead of seeking to give your daughters a musical education, instruct them in these useful branches which have the closest connection with life and health. Teach them all the mysteries of cooking. Show them that this is a part of their education and essential for them in order to become Christians. Unless the food is prepared in a wholesome, palatable manner, it cannot be converted into good blood to build up the wasting tissues. Your daughters may love music, and this may be all right; it may add to the happiness of the family; but the knowledge of music without the knowledge of cookery is not worth much. When your daughters have families of their own, an understanding of music and fancy work will not provide for the table a well cooked dinner, prepared with nicety, so that they will not blush to place it before their most-esteemed friends. Mothers, yours is a sacred work. May God help you to take it up with His glory in view and work earnestly, patiently, and lovingly for the present and future good of your children, having an eye single to the glory of God.

284. The proper cooking of food is an essential requirement, especially when meat is not served.

Healthful Living, 76.

THE proper cooking of food is a most essential requirement, especially where meat is not made an article of diet. Something must be prepared to take the place of meat, and these foods must be well prepared, so that meat will not be desired.

285. Health reformers especially should be good cooks for their own benefit, but also in order to teach others.

Healthful Living, 77.

YOU profess to be health reformers, and for this very reason you should become good cooks. Those who can avail themselves of the advantages of properly conducted hygienic cooking-schools, will find it a great benefit, both in their own practice and in teaching others. . . . One reason why many have become discouraged in practicing health reform is that they have not learned how to cook so that proper food, simply prepared, would supply the place of the diet to which they have been accustomed.

286. Many need cooking classes, for they know not how to prepare simple and appetizing dishes.

Healthful Living, 77.

WE NEED persons who will educate themselves to cook healthfully. Many know how to cook meats and vegetables in different forms, yet do not understand how to prepare simple and appetizing dishes.

287. We must first eat properly, and then we can live properly.

Healthful Living, 76.

THOSE who will not eat and drink from principle, will not be governed by principle in other things.

288. Christ gave an example of how to eat properly when invited out.

Manuscript Releases, vol. 7, 412

WHILE Christ accepted invitations to feasts and gatherings, He did not partake of all the food offered Him, but quietly ate of that which was appropriate for His physical necessities, avoiding the many things that He did not need. His disciples were frequently invited with Him, and His conduct was a lesson to them, teaching them not to indulge appetite by overeating or by eating improper food. He showed them that portions of the food provided could be passed by, and portions chosen.

Christ went to these feasts because He wished to show those who were excluding themselves from the society of their fellow men, how wrong their course of action was. He wished to teach them that truth was given to be imparted to those who had it not. If they had truth, why keep it selfishly to themselves. The world is perishing for want of the living Truth.

The True Remedies—VII
Water

See also paragraph numbers 242 & 243.

289. Pure water is one of Heaven's choicest blessings to assist us in maintaining our health and to recover it if we are ill.

Counsels on Diet and Foods, 419.

IN HEALTH and in sickness, pure water is one of Heaven's choicest blessings. Its proper use promotes health. It is the beverage which God provided to quench the thirst of animals and man. Drunk freely, it helps to supply the necessities of the system, and assists nature to resist disease.

290. Pure water and fresh air invigorate the vital organs, helping nature to overcome disease.

Healthful Living, 187.

PURE water to drink and fresh air to breathe invigorate the vital organs, purify the blood, and help nature in her task of overcoming the bad conditions of the system.

291. Hot drinks may be beneficial as a medicine, but large quantities of hot food or drink enfeeble the body.

Counsels on Diet and Foods, 106.

HOT drinks are not required, except as a medicine. The stomach is greatly injured by a large quantity of hot food and hot drink. Thus the throat and digestive organs, and through them the other organs of the body, are enfeebled.

292. A pint of hot water taken before meals can help relieve suffering.

Counsels on Diet and Foods, 419.

WATER can be used in many ways to relieve suffering. Drafts of clear, hot water taken before eating (half quart. more or less), will never do any harm, but will rather be productive of good.

293. A brief, total fast, except for pure, soft water, will many times be beneficial.

Healthful Living, 226.

FAST for one or two meals, and drink only pure, soft water. The loss of a meal or two will enable the overburdened system to overcome slight indispositions; and even graver difficulties may sometimes be overcome by this simple process.

294. Soft water is recommended for bathing as well as for drinking purposes.

Healthful Living, 226.

IF THEY would become enlightened. . . . and accustom themselves to outdoor exercise, and to air in their houses, summer and winter, and use soft water for drinking and bathing purposes, they would be comparatively well and happy, instead of dragging out a miserable existence.

295. The use of pure, soft water for the cleansing of the skin and the clothes is an important aspect of preventing disease.

Selected Messages, book 2, 460.

A GREAT amount of suffering might be saved if all would labor to prevent disease, by strictly obeying the laws of health. Strict habits of cleanliness should be observed. Many, while well, will not take the trouble to keep in a healthy condition. They neglect personal cleanliness, and are not careful to keep their clothing pure. Impurities are constantly and imperceptibly passing from the body, through the pores, and if the surface of the skin is not kept in a healthy condition, the system is burdened with impure matter. If the clothing worn is not often washed, and frequently aired, it becomes filthy with impurities which are thrown off from the body by sensible and insensible perspiration. And if the garments worn are not frequently cleansed from these impurities, the pores of the skin absorb again the waste matter thrown off. The impurities of the body, if not allowed to escape, are taken back into the blood, and forced upon the internal organs. Nature, to relieve herself of poisonous impurities, makes an effort to free the system, which effort produces fevers, and what is termed disease. But even then, if those who are afflicted would assist nature in her efforts, by the use of pure, soft water, much suffering would be prevented. But many, instead of doing this, and seeking to remove the poisonous matter from the system, take a more deadly poison into the system, to remove a poison already there.

296. Dirty clothes permit the reabsorption of waste materials.

The Ministry of Healing, 276.

IT IS important also that the clothing be kept clean. The garments worn absorb the waste matter that passes off through the pores; if they are not frequently changed and washed, the impurities will be reabsorbed.

297. By improving the circulation a daily bath helps prevent colds and improves the function of many organs.

The Ministry of Healing, 276.

MOST persons would receive benefit from a cool or tepid bath every day, morning or evening. Instead of increasing the liability to take cold, a bath, properly taken, fortifies against cold, because it improves the circulation; the blood is brought to the surface, and a more easy and regular flow is obtained. The mind and the body are alike invigorated. The muscles become more flexible, the intellect is made brighter. The bath is a soother of the nerves. Bathing helps the bowels, the stomach, and the liver, giving health and energy to each, and it promotes digestion.

298. A bath, properly taken, relieves congestion and improves the blood flow through all of the vessels.

Healthful Living, 228.

WHETHER a person is sick or well, respiration is more free and easy if bathing is practiced. By it the muscles become more flexible, the body and mind are alike invigorated, the intellect is made brighter, and every faculty becomes livelier. The bath is a soother of the nerves. It promotes general perspiration, quickens the circulation, overcomes obstructions in the system, and acts beneficially on the kidneys and the urinary organs. Bathing helps the bowel, stomach, and liver, giving energy and new life to each. It also promotes digestion, and instead of the system being weakened, it is strengthened. Instead of increasing the liability to cold, a bath, properly taken, fortifies against cold, because the circulation is improved, and the uterine organs, which are more or less congested, are relieved; for the blood is brought to the surface, and more easy and regular flow of the blood through all the blood vessels is obtained.

299. Bathing cleanses the skin and keeps it moist and supple, thus improving the circulation.

Healthful Living, 187.

BATHING frees the skin from the accumulation of impurities which are constantly collecting, and keeps the skin moist and supple, thereby increasing and equalizing the circulation.

300. Water, without a proper diet, benefits the patient little.

Healthful Living, 226.

THE use of water can accomplish but little if the patient does not feel the necessity of also strictly attending to his diet.

301. Healthy individuals, as well as the sick, should bathe at least twice a week.

Healthful Living, 227.

PERSONS in health should . . . by all means bathe as often as twice a week. Those who are not in health have impurities of the blood. . . . The skin needs to be carefully and thoroughly cleansed, that the pores may do their work in freeing the body from impurities; therefore feeble persons who are diseased surely need the advantages and blessings of bathing as often as twice a week, and frequently even more than this is positively necessary.

302. Rubbing after a bath until the skin glows also improves the circulation.

Healthful Living, 192.

TWICE a week she should take a general bath, as cool as will be agreeable, a little cooler every time, until the skin is toned up.

Upon rising in the morning, most persons would be benefited by taking a sponge bath, or, if more agreeable, a hand bath, with merely a washbowl of water; this will remove impurities from the skin.

Frequent bathing is very beneficial, especially at night just before retiring, or upon rising in the morning. It will take but a few moments to give the children a bath, and to rub them until their bodies are in a glow. This brings the blood to the surface, relieving the brain. Bathe frequently in pure soft water, followed by gentle rubbing.

303. The intelligent use of water, internally and externally, will help quench the flame of fever cases.

Healthful Living, 227.

REDUCE the feverish state of the system by a careful and intelligent application of water.

If, in their fevered state, water had been given them to drink freely, and applications had also been made externally, long days and nights of suffering would have been saved, and many precious lives spared.

The fire of fever seems consuming him. He longs for pure water to moisten the parched lips, to quench the raging thirst, and to cool the fevered brow. . . . The blessed, heaven-sent water, skillfully applied, would quench the devouring flame.

304. None are excused for lack of knowledge or interest in the uses of water for simple home treatments.

The Ministry of Healing, 237.

THE external application of water is one of the easiest and most satisfactory ways of regulating the circulation of the blood. A cold or cool bath is an excellent tonic. Warm baths open the pores and thus aid in the elimination of impurities. Both warm and neutral baths soothe the nerves and equalize the circulation. But many have never learned by experience the beneficial effects of the proper use of water, and they are afraid of it. Water treatments are not appreciated as they should be, and to apply them skillfully requires work that many are unwilling to perform. But none should feel excused for ignorance or indifference on this subject. There are many ways in which water can be applied to relieve pain and check disease. All should become intelligent in its use in simple home treatments. Mothers, especially, should know how to care for their families in both health and sickness.

The True Remedies—VIII
Trust In Divine Power

305. We are to understand each of our body's organs and to realize that they are to be servants to the mind, which is the capital of the body.

Testimonies, vol. 3, 136.

TO BECOME acquainted with the wonderful human organism, the bones, muscles, stomach, liver, bowels, heart, and pores of the skin, and to understand the dependence of one organ upon another for the healthful action of all, is a study in which most mothers take no interest. They know nothing of the influence of the body upon the mind and of the mind upon the body. The mind, which allies finite to the infinite, they do not seem to understand. Every organ of the body was made to be servant to the mind. The mind is the capital of the body.

306. It is through the mind, or brain nerves, that Heaven communicates with us and transforms us.

Testimonies, vol. 2, 347.

THE brain nerves which communicate with the entire system are the only medium through which Heaven can communicate to man and affect his inmost life.

Spirit of Prophecy, vol. 2, 129.

THE mind is an invisible agent of God to produce tangible results. Its influence is powerful, and governs the actions of men. If purified from all evil, it is the motive power of good. The regenerating Spirit of God, taking possession of the mind, transforms the life; wicked thoughts are put away, evil deeds are renounced, love, peace, and humility take the place of anger, envy, and strife. That power which no human eye can see, has created a new being in the image of God.

Trust In Your Creator

307. We and all things existing were created by the spoken word of the Lord Jehovah.

The Ministry of Healing, 414–415.

IN THE creation of the earth, God was not indebted to preexisting matter. "He spake, and it was; . . . He commanded, and it stood fast." Psalm 33:9. All things, material or spiritual, stood up before the Lord Jehovah at His voice and were created for His own purpose. The heavens and all the host of them, the earth and all things therein, came into existence by the breath of His mouth.

In the creation of man was manifest the agency of a personal God. When God had made man in His image, the human form was perfect in all its arrangements, but it was without life. Then a personal, self-existing God breathed into that form the breath of life, and man became a living, intelligent being. All parts of the human organism were set in action.

The heart, the arteries, the veins, the tongue, the hands, the feet, the senses, the faculties of the mind, all began their work, and all were placed under law. Man became a living soul. Through Christ the Word, a personal God created man and endowed him with intelligence and power. . . .

Above all lower orders of being, God designed that man, the crowning work of His creation, should express His thought and reveal His glory.

308. God created man out of the dust of the earth in His likeness and gave him dominion over the earth.

Patriarchs and Prophets, 44–45.

AFTER the earth with its teeming animal and vegetable life had been called into existence, man, the crowning work of the Creator, and the one for whom the beautiful earth had been fitted up, was brought upon the stage of action. To him was given dominion over all that his eye could behold; for "God said, Let Us make man in Our image, after Our likeness: and let them have dominion over . . . all the earth. . . . So God created man in His own image; . . . male and female created He them." Here is clearly set forth the origin of the human race; and the divine record is so plainly stated that there is no occasion for erroneous conclusions. God created man in His own image. Here is no mystery. There is no ground for the supposition that man was evolved by slow degrees of development from the lower forms of animal or vegetable life. Such teaching lowers the great work of the Creator to the level of man's narrow, earthly conceptions. Men are so intent upon excluding God from the sovereignty of the universe that they degrade man and defraud him of the dignity of his origin. He who set the starry worlds on high and tinted with delicate skill the flowers of the field, who filled the earth and the heavens with the wonders of His power, when He came to crown His glorious work, to place one in the midst to stand as ruler of the fair earth, did not fail to create a being worthy of the hand that gave him life. The genealogy of our race, as given by inspiration, traces back its origin, not to a line of developing germs, mollusks, and quadrupeds, but to the great Creator. Though formed from the dust, Adam was "the son of God."

Trust In Your Sustainer

309. Every mechanism of our bodies is kept in order and activity by the power of an ever-present God.

The Ministry of Healing, 417.

THE mechanism of the human body cannot be fully understood; it presents mysteries that baffle the most intelligent. It is not as the result of a mechanism, which, once set in motion, continues its work, that the pulse beats and breath follows breath. In God we live and move and have our being. The beating heart, the throbbing pulse, every nerve and muscle in the living organism, is kept in order and activity by the power of an ever-present God.

Manuscript Releases, vol. 3, 329.

YOUR heart beats on. On that pulsation depends your life. Its beating is independent of your will. You eat and sleep in careless indifference. But God's guardian care over you is unceasing. He controls the ebb and flow of the vital current. Where is your gratitude that should rise from human lips for His preserving care?

310. Christ sustains us hour by hour and moment by moment.

Education, 97–198.

NOT only is He the originator of all, but He is the life of everything that lives. It is His life that we receive in the sunshine, in the pure, sweet air, in food which builds up our bodies and sustains our strength. It is by His life that we exist, hour by hour, moment by moment.

311. Saint and sinner alike are constantly maintained in this temporal life by the death of Christ in our stead on the cross.

The Desire of Ages, 660.

TO THE death of Christ we owe even this earthly life. The bread we eat is the purchase of His broken body. The water we drink is bought by His spilled blood. Never one, saint or sinner, eats his daily food, but he is nourished by the body and the blood of Christ. The cross of Calvary is stamped on every loaf. It is reflected in every water spring.

312. Only through a life in harmony with the Creator's can we be restored to the original, sinless harmony of His universe.

Medical Ministry, 10.

THE same power that upholds nature is working also in man. The same great laws that guide alike the star and the atom control human life. The laws that govern the heart's action, regulating the flow of the current of life to the body, are the laws of the mighty Intelligence that has the jurisdiction of the soul. From Him all life proceeds. Only in harmony with Him can be found its true sphere of action. For all the objects of His creation the condition is the same—a life sustained by receiving the life of God, a life exercised in harmony with the Creator's will. To transgress His law, physical, mental, or moral, is to place one's self out of harmony with the universe, to introduce discord, anarchy, ruin.

313. God upholds and sustains His creation by working through His own laws of nature.

The Ministry of Healing, 416.

GOD is constantly employed in upholding and using as His servants the things that He has made. He works through the laws of nature, using them as His instruments. They are not self-acting. Nature in her work testifies of the intelligent presence and active agency of a Being who moves in all things according to His will.

Trust In Your Partner

314. God is our Partner in temporal matters as well as in all spiritual achievements.

Review and Herald, May 28, 1908.

GOD has originated and proclaimed the principles on which divine and human agencies are to combine in temporal matters as well as all spiritual achievements. They are to be linked together in all human pursuits, in mechanical and agricultural labor, in mercantile and scientific enterprises. In all lines of work it is necessary that there be cooperation between God and man. God has provided facilities with which to enrich and beautify the earth. But the strength and ingenuity of human agencies are required to make the very best use of the material. God had filled the earth with treasure, but the gold and silver are hidden in the earth, and the exercise of man's powers is required to secure this treasure which God has provided. Man's energy and tact are to be used in connection with the power of God in bringing the gold and silver from the mines, and trees from the forest. But unless by his miracle-working power God cooperated with man, enabling him to use his physical and mental capabilities, the treasures in our world would be useless.

315. Every human being is to work together with God in all useful employment.

Review and Herald, May 28, 1908.

GOD desires every human being in our world to be a worker together with him. This is the lesson we are to learn from all useful employment, making homes in the forest, felling trees to build houses, clearing land for cultivation. God has provided the wood and the land, and to man he has given the work of putting them in such shape that they will be a blessing. In this work man is wholly dependent upon God. The fitting of the ships that cross the broad ocean is not alone due to the talent and ingenuity of the human agent. God is the great Architect. Without his cooperation, without the aid of the higher intelligences, how worthless would be the plans of men. God must aid, else every device is worthless.

Trust In Your Healer

316. Whenever health is restored, it is through the direct power of God; for He is the great Healer.

Medical Ministry, 11–12.

GOD'S healing power runs all through nature. If a human being cuts his flesh or breaks a bone, nature at once begins to heal the injury, and thus preserve the man's life. But man can place himself in a position where nature is trammeled so that she cannot do her work. . . . If tobacco is used, . . . the healing power of nature is weakened to a greater or less extent. . . . When intoxicating liquor is used, the system is not able to resist disease in its original God-given power as a healer. It is God who has made the provision that nature shall work to restore the exhausted powers. The power is of God. He is the great Healer.

317. Christ's miracles were a manifestation of His

constant work to heal us; for He is the Restorer, while Satan is the destroyer.

The Ministry of Healing, 112–113.

THE Saviour in His miracles revealed the power that is continually at work in man's behalf, to sustain and to heal him. Through the agencies of nature, God is working, day by day, hour by hour, moment by moment, to keep us alive, to build up and restore us. When any part of the body sustains injury, a healing process is at once begun; nature's agencies are set at work to restore soundness. But the power working through these agencies is the power of God. All life-giving power is from Him. When one recovers from disease, it is God who restores him.

Sickness, suffering, and death are work of an antagonistic power. Satan is the destroyer; God is the restorer.

318. Many will be healed miraculously, while many others will be healed by the same power through the slower working of natural law.

Manuscript Releases, vol. 9, 287.

MANY who are threatened with consumption will be healed through faith. Many others will be healed through proper eating and drinking and through living largely in the open air.

319. We ask for a miracle and God directs us to His simple, natural remedies that are within our reach.

The Seventh-day Adventist Bible Commentary, vol. 7, 938.

GOD'S miracles do not always bear the outward semblance of miracles. Often they are brought about in a way which looks like the natural course of events. When we pray for the sick, we also work for them. We answer our own prayers by using the remedies within our reach. Water, wisely applied, is a most powerful remedy. As it is used intelligently, favorable results are seen. God has given us intelligence, and He desires us to make the most of His health-giving blessings. . . . We are to use every blessing God has placed within our reach for the deliverance of those in danger.

Natural means, used in accordance with God's will, bring about supernatural results. We ask for a miracle, and the Lord directs the mind to some simple remedy.

320. We are to show our faith in God's healing power by placing ourselves in the condition most favorable to recovery.

Spalding and Magan, 7.

I THANK the Lord that it is our privilege to cooperate with Him in the work of restoration, availing ourselves of all possible advantages in the recovery of health. It is no denial of our faith to place ourselves in the condition most favorable to recovery.

Trust In Your Pardoner

321. What many of the ill most need is relief from the burden of guilt that only a healing of the sin-sick soul by Christ can provide.

Testimonies, vol. 4, 579.

MANY are suffering from maladies of the soul far more than from diseases of the body, and they will find no relief until they shall come to Christ, the wellspring of life. Complaints of weariness, loneliness, and dissatisfaction will then cease. Satisfying joys will give vigor to the mind and health and vital energy to the body.

The burden of sin, with its unrest and unsatisfied desires, lies at the very foundation of a large share of the maladies the sinner suffers. Christ is the mighty healer of the sin-sick soul. These poor afflicted ones need to have a clearer knowledge of Him whom to know aright is life eternal. They need to be patiently and kindly yet earnestly taught how to throw open the windows of the soul and let the sunlight of God's love come in to illuminate the darkened chambers of the mind.

322. Sickness of the mind is the foundation of ninety percent of man's ills, and the religion of Christ is its most effectual remedy.

Testimonies, vol. 5, 443–444.

SATAN is the originator of disease; and the physician is warring against his work and power. Sickness of the mind prevails everywhere. Nine tenths of the diseases from which men suffer have their foundation here. Perhaps some living home trouble is, like a canker, eating to the very soul and weakening the life forces. Remorse for sin sometimes undermines the constitution and unbalances the mind. There are erroneous doctrines also, as that of an eternally burning hell and the endless torment of the wicked, that, by giving exaggerated and distorted views of the character of God, have produced the same result upon sensitive minds. Infidels have made the most of these unfortunate cases, attributing insanity to religion; but this is a gross libel and one which they will not be pleased to meet by and by. The religion of Christ, so far from being the cause of insanity, is one of its most effectual remedies; for it is a potent soother of the nerves.

Trust In Your Enabler

323. We can live in harmony with God's will only as we surrender our will to His will and His enabling power.

The Ministry of Healing, 176.

THE tempted one needs to understand the true force of the will. This is the governing power in the nature of man the power of decision, of choice. Everything depends on the right action of the will. Desires for goodness and purity are right, so far as they go; but if we stop here, they avail nothing. Many will go down to ruin while hoping and desiring to overcome their propensities. They do not yield the will to God. They do not choose to serve Him.

God has given us the power of choice; it is ours to exercise. We cannot change our hearts, we cannot control our thoughts, our impulses, our affections. We cannot make ourselves pure, fit for God's service. But we can choose to serve God, we can give Him our will; then He will work in us to will and to do according to His good pleasure. Thus our whole nature will be brought under the control of Christ.

Through the right exercise of the will, an entire change may be made in the life. By yielding up the will to Christ, we ally ourselves with divine power. We receive strength from above to hold us steadfast. A pure and noble life, a life of victory over appetite and lust, is possible to everyone who will unite his weak, wavering human will to the omnipotent, unwavering will of God.

324. We have a much greater need than previous generations for God's enabling power to overcome perverted appetite.

Testimonies, vol. 3, 488.

THE necessity for the men of this generation to call to their aid the power of the will, strengthened by the grace of God, in order to withstand the temptations of Satan and resist the least indulgence of perverted appetite is twice as great as it was several generations ago. But the present generation have less power of self-control than had those who lived then. . . .

The Redeemer of the world came from heaven to help man in his weakness, that, in the power which Jesus came to bring him, he might become strong to overcome appetite and passion, and might be victor on every point.

Trust In Your Redeemer

325. When we accept Christ as our Redeemer and cease from our rebellion, He then bestows upon us His infinite treasures.

Christ's Object Lessons, 119–120.

IN CHRIST'S day many heard the gospel, but their minds were darkened by false teaching, and they did not recognize in the humble Teacher of Galilee the Sent of God. But after Christ's ascension His enthronement in His mediatorial kingdom was signalized by the outpouring of the Holy Spirit. On the day of Pentecost the Spirit was given. Christ's witnesses proclaimed the power of the risen Saviour. The light of heaven penetrated the darkened minds of those who had been deceived by the enemies of Christ. They now saw Him exalted to be "a Prince and a Saviour, for to give repentance of Israel, and forgiveness of sins." Acts 5:31. They saw Him encircled with the glory of heaven, with infinite treasures in His hands to bestow upon all who would turn from their rebellion. As the apostles set forth the glory of the Only-Begotten of the Father, three thousand souls were convicted. They were made to see themselves as they were, sinful and polluted, and Christ as their friend and Redeemer. Christ was lifted up, Christ was glorified, through the power of the Holy Spirit resting upon men. By faith these believers saw Him as the One who had borne humiliation, suffering, and death that they might not perish but have everlasting life. The revelation of Christ by the Spirit brought to them a realizing sense of His power and majesty, and they stretched forth their hands to Him by faith, saying, "I believe."

326. We can be cleansed and saved from disobedience only as we behold and accept His love as shown through His blood shed for us on the cross.

The Seventh-day Adventist Bible Commentary, vol. 5, 1132–1133.

THE plan of salvation, making manifest the justice and love of God, provides an eternal safeguard against defection in unfallen worlds, as well as among those who shall be redeemed by the blood of the Lamb. Our only hope is perfect trust in the blood of Him who can save to the uttermost all that come unto God by Him. The death of Christ on the cross of Calvary is our only hope in this world, and it will be our theme in the world to come. . . . Why should man not study the theme of redemption? It is the greatest subject that can engage the human mind. If men would contemplate the love of Christ, displayed in the cross, their faith would be strengthened to appropriate the merits of His shed blood, and they would be cleansed and saved from sin.

Trust In Your Restorer

327. When we trust Christ as our Creator, our Sustainer, our Healer, our Enabler, our Pardoner, and our Redeemer, then He also becomes our Restorer to His eternal Eden.

The Great Controversy, 673–674.

THE time has come to which holy men have looked with longing since the flaming sword barred the first pair from Eden, the time for "the redemption of the purchased possession." Ephesians 1:14. The earth originally given to man as his kingdom, betrayed by him into the hands of Satan, and so long held by the mighty foe, has been brought back by the great plan of redemption. All that was lost by sin has been restored. "Thus saith the Lord . . . that formed the earth and made it; He hath established it, He created it not in vain, He formed it to be inhabited." Isaiah 45:18. God's original purpose in the creation of the earth is fulfilled as it is made the eternal abode of the redeemed. "The righteous shall inherit the land, and dwell therein forever." Psalm 37:29.

A fear of making the future inheritance seem too material has led many to spiritualize away the very truths which lead us to look upon it as our home. Christ assured His disciples that He went to prepare mansions for them in the Father's house. Those who accept the teachings of God's word will not be wholly ignorant concerning the heavenly abode. And yet, "eye hath not seen, nor ear heard, neither have entered into the heart of man, the things which God hath prepared for them that love Him." 1Cor. 2:9. Human language is inadequate to describe the reward of the righteous. It will be known only to those who behold it. No finite mind can comprehend the glory of the Paradise of God.

In the Bible the inheritance of the saved is called "a country." Hebrews 11:14–16. There the heavenly Shepherd leads His flock to fountains of living water. The tree of life yields its fruit every month, and the leaves of the tree are for the service of the nations. There are ever-flowing streams, clear as crystal, and beside them waving trees cast their shadows upon the paths prepared for the ransomed of the Lord. There the wide-spreading plains swell into hills of beauty, and the mountains of God rear their lofty summits. On those peaceful plains, beside those living streams, God's people, so long pilgrims and wanderers, shall find a home.

The Lord's Work

328. Every self-sacrificing worker is to do the Lord's work of loving ministry.

Review and Herald, vol. 4, 387.

THE Lord continually performed deeds of loving ministry, and this every minister of the gospel should do. He has appointed us to be His ambassadors, to carry forward *His work* in the world. To every true, self-sacrificing worker is given the commission, "Go ye into all the world, and preach the gospel to every creature." (emphasis supplied).

329. We are to follow the example of Christ's work upon this earth.

Review and Herald, vol. 4, 387.

READ carefully the instruction given in the New Testament. The work that the Great Teacher did in connection with His disciples is the example we are to follow.

330. Christ gave His whole earthly life to teach us how to work for God.

Battle Creek Letters, 113.

THE great Teacher, while on this earth, gave His whole life to teach us how to work as devoted, consecrated missionaries for God.

331. Christ's teaching, healing, and preaching is the work outlined for those who have greater truth than any previous generation.

Australasian Record, 119.

CHRIST is our example. Of His work we read, Jesus went about all Galilee, teaching in their synagogues, and preaching the gospel of the kingdom, and healing all manner of sickness and all manner of disease among the people. They brought unto Him all sick people that were taken with divers diseases and torments, and those which were possessed with devils, and those which were lunatic, and those that had the palsy, and He healed them.

Christ healed the people, and then to those whom He healed and to those who had witnessed His healing, He preached the gospel of the kingdom. This is *the work* outlined before those who have in trust the greatest wealth of truth ever committed to mortals. (emphasis supplied).

332. The true gospel consists of Christlike work for both the body and the soul.

My Life Today, 224.

THE union of Christlike work for the body and Christlike work for the soul is the true interpretation of the gospel.

333. Like Christ, the apostles, and the seventy we are to unite medical missionary work with the ministry of the Word.

Counsels on Health, 517.

IN ALL His labors He united the medical missionary work with the ministry of the Word. He sent out the twelve apostles and afterward the seventy, to preach the gospel to the people, and He gave them power also to heal the sick and to cast out devils in His name. Thus should the Lord's messengers enter His work today.

334. Christ united healing and teaching; but He spent the most time in healing, and He is our Example.

The Gospel Herald, 137.

THE Lord Jesus is our Example. He came to the world as a servant of mankind. He went from city to city, from village to village, teaching the gospel of the kingdom, and healing the sick. Christ spent more time in healing than in teaching. As our example, Christ linked closely together the work of healing and teaching, and in this our day they should not be separated.

335. The ministry of the Word and the healing of the sick are one work, and they never can and never will be separated.

Special Testimonies, Series B, 256.

THE Holy Spirit never has, and never will in the future, divorce the medical missionary work from the gospel ministry. They cannot be divorced. Bound up with Jesus Christ, the ministry of the Word and the healing of the sick are one.

336. Ministers are to work for the body as well as for the soul, taking the people right where they are and helping them in every way possible.

Review and Herald, vol. 4, 372.

TO TAKE people right where they are, whatever their position or condition, and help them in every way possible this is gospel ministry. Those who are diseased in body are nearly always diseased in mind, and when the soul is sick, the body also is affected. Ministers should feel it a part of their work to minister to the sick and afflicted whenever opportunity presents itself. The minister of the gospel is to present the message, which must be received if the people are to become sanctified and made ready for the coming of the Lord. This work is to embrace all that was embraced in Christ's ministry.

337. The gospel ministry is a union of the medical missionary work and the ministry of the Word.

Review and Herald, vol. 4, 372.

The Final Work

THE gospel ministry is an organization for the proclamation of the truth to the sick and to the well. It combines the medical missionary work and the ministry of the Word. By these combined agencies, opportunities are given to communicate light, and to present the gospel to all classes and all grades of society. God wants the ministers and the church members to take a decided, active interest in the medical missionary work.

338. Christ left His ministry of healing to His followers with instructions to carry it to the whole world.

Battle Creek Letters, 113.

WHEN Jesus was about to ascend to His Father, He gave His ministry of healing to His followers, leaving with them the commission, "Go ye therefore and teach all nations, baptizing them in the name of the Father, and of the Son, and of the Holy Ghost; teaching them to observe all things whatsoever I have commanded you; and, lo, I am with you alway, even unto the end of the world."

339. Those who believe in Jesus Christ are to be co-workers with Him, revealing in word and deed a representation of His love.

Pacific Union Recorder, 1.

ONE who believes in Jesus Christ as a personal Saviour is to be a co-worker with Him, bound up with His heart of infinite love, cooperating with Him in works of self-denial and benevolence. Christ has withdrawn Himself from the earth, but His followers are still left in the world. And they are to give in word and action, and in their unselfish benevolence, a representation of Christ's love.

340. Christ is the pattern Man, the great Medical Missionary, and we are to do the same self-sacrificial work.

Loma Linda Messages, 61.

CHRIST stands before us as the pattern Man, the great Medical Missionary an example for all who should come after. His love, pure and holy, blessed all who came within the sphere of its influence. His character was absolutely perfect, free from the slightest stain of sin. He came as an expression of the perfect love of God, not to crush, not to judge and condemn, but to heal every weak, defective character, to save men and women from Satan's power. . . . What, then, is the example that we are to set to the world? We are to do the same work that the great Medical Missionary undertook in our behalf. We are to follow the path of self-sacrifice trodden by Christ.

341. Medical missionary work combines teaching and healing, and today we are to follow Christ's example in uniting them.

Loma Linda Messages, 338.

CHRIST, the great Medical Missionary, is our example. Of Him it is written, that "He went about all Galilee, teaching in their synagogues, and preaching the gospel of the kingdom, and healing all manner sickness and diseases among the people." He healed the sick, and preached the gospel. In His service, healing and teaching were linked closely together. Today they are not to be separated.

342. Connected with the Divine Healer and uniting His healing power with the gospel message, we will have success in sharing the power of God unto salvation.

Loma Linda Messages, 338.

CHRIST understood the work that needed to be done for suffering humanity. As He was sending out the twelve disciples on their first missionary tour, He said to them, "As ye go, preach, saying, The kingdom of heaven is at hand. Heal the sick, cleanse the lepers, raise the dead, cast out devils; freely ye have received, freely give." The fulfillment of this commission by the disciples made their message the power of God unto salvation.

It is the divine plan that we shall work as the disciples worked. Connected with the Divine Healer, we may do great good in the world. The gospel is the only antidote for sin. As Christ's witnesses we are to bear testimony to its power. We are to bring the afflicted ones to the Saviour. His transforming grace and miracle-working power will win many souls to the truth. His healing power, united with the gospel message, will bring us success in emergencies. The Holy Spirit will work upon hearts, and we shall see the salvation of God.

343. We must not follow Satan's schemes to separate the medical missionary work from the work of the gospel ministry.

Loma Linda Messages, 339.

THE medical missionary work is not to be carried forward as something apart from the work of the gospel ministry. The Lord's people are to be one. There is to be no separation in His work. . . . The two lines of work must not be separated. Satan will invent every possible scheme to separate those whom God is seeking to make one. We must not be misled by his devices. The medical missionary work is to be connected with the work of the third angel's message, as the hand is connected with the body.

344. Every medical practitioner is to know how to heal sin-sick souls, as well as how to heal bodily disease.

Medical Ministry, 31.

EVERY medical practitioner, whether he acknowledges it or not, is responsible for the souls as well as the bodies of his patients. The Lord expects of us much more than we often do for Him. Every physician should be a devoted, intelligent, gospel medical missionary, familiar with Heaven's remedy for the sin-sick soul, as well as with the science of healing bodily disease.

345. Nurses are to unite the teaching of the gospel with the work of healing.

The Gospel Herald, 137.

IN OUR schools and sanitariums nurses should be trained to go out as medical missionary evangelists. They should unite the teaching of the gospel of Christ with the work of healing.

346. Our ministers would be far better able to do the

work of Christ if they were educated in medical missionary lines.

Medical Ministry, 239.

IF OUR ministers would work earnestly to obtain an education in medical missionary lines they would be far better fitted to do the work Christ did as a medical missionary. By diligent study and practice, they can become so well acquainted with the principles of health reform, that wherever they go they will be a great blessing to the people they meet.

347. Canvassers should learn how to treat disease.

Medical Ministry, 249.

IT IS medical missionaries that are needed all through the field. Canvassers should improve every opportunity granted them to learn how to treat disease.

348. Every worker should do what he can in the treatment of disease.

Pacific Union Recorder, 3.

LET each worker put into practice what he knows regarding the treatment of disease. Thus suffering may be relieved, and opportunities will be found to break the bread of life to starving souls.

349. Students are to receive practical instruction in how to teach cooking and how to care for the sick.

Spalding and Magan, 126.

IT IS essential that students be taught how to do missionary work, not only by pen and voice, but by working with them in various missionary lines. All about us there are persons who need to be taught how to cook and how to treat the sick. By engaging in these lines of work we practice the truth as it is in Jesus. Teachers and students need to study how to engage in this work. The teachers should take students to places where help is needed, giving them practical instruction in how to care for the sick.

350. Parents should not let children or home duties be an excuse not to do medical missionary work.

Review and Herald, vol. 4, 439.

ALL can do something. In an effort to excuse themselves, some say, "My home duties, my children, claim my time and my means." Parents, your children should be your helping hand, increasing your power and ability to work for the Master. Children are the younger members of the Lord's family. They should be led to consecrate themselves to God, whose they are by creation and by redemption. They should be taught that all their powers of body, mind, and soul are His. They should be trained to help in various kinds of unselfish service. Do not allow your children to be hindrances. With you the children should share spiritual as well as physical burdens. By helping others they increase their own happiness and usefulness.

351. Idle children are to be instructed, so that they may become workers in the army of medical missionaries.

Battle Creek Letters, 26.

THE medical missionary work is to burst all barriers. All are invited to take a part in it, and help where help is needed. The wealthy are to be reached, and their sympathy and assistance solicited; for are they not the Lord's stewards? Idle children are to be instructed; they are to enlist in the army of workers to help the sick and suffering. Train the children, for they are the Lord's heritage.

352. Unlearned men are often chosen of God to do a special work in medical missionary lines.

Testimonies, vol. 7, 25–26.

THOSE whom God chooses as workers are not always talented, in the estimation of the world. Sometimes He selects unlearned men. To those He gives a special work. They reach a class to whom others could not obtain access. Opening the heart to the truth, they are made wise in and through Christ. Their lives inhale and exhale the fragrance of godliness. Their words are thoughtfully considered before they are spoken. They strive to promote the well-being of their fellow men. They take relief and happiness to the needy and distressed. They realize the necessity of ever remaining under Christ's training, that they may work in harmony with God's will. They study how best to follow the Saviour's example of cross bearing and self-denial. They are God's witnesses, revealing His compassion and love, and ascribing all the glory to Him whom they love and serve.

353. Those with only one talent are called to do what they can to roll back the wave of disease and suffering.

Loma Linda Messages, 72A

THE Lord desires every one to do his best. You may think that you can do very little; but remember that in the parable of the talents, Christ did not represent all the servants as receiving the same amount. To one servant was given five talents; to another, two, and to still another, one. If you have but one talent, use it wisely, increasing it by putting it out to the exchangers. Do what you can to roll back the wave of disease and suffering that is sweeping over our world. Come up to the help of the Lord, to the help of the Lord against the mighty powers of darkness.

354. Every man is called to assist the great Medical Missionary Worker in the highways and byways.

The Paulson Collection, 15–16.

GOD calls upon every man to cooperate with the great Medical Missionary Worker, and to go forth into the highways and byways.

355. Every true believer will follow the Saviour's example in doing medical missionary work.

Review and Herald, vol. 5, 50.

THE Saviour lived on this earth a life that love for God will constrain every true believer in Christ to live. Following His example, in our medical missionary work we shall reveal to the world that we are His representatives and that our credentials are from above.

356. At baptism every one of us was set apart to follow Christ in being a healing missionary.

Review and Herald, vol. 4, 369.

THE Lord wants every one of us to educate himself for God. At baptism, in the name of the Father, and of the Son, and of the Holy Ghost we were set apart to engage in the very work that Christ came to the world to do. What was He? In the highest sense He was a missionary, and He was a healing missionary.

357. Our duty to minister to the sick cannot be done for us by others.

Review and Herald, vol. 6, 244.

CHRIST commits to His followers an individual work a work that cannot be done by proxy. Ministry to the sick and the poor, the giving of the gospel to the lost, is not to be left to committees or organized charities. Individual responsibility, individual effort, personal sacrifice, is the requirement of the gospel.

358. The giving of our means to do the Lord's work will not take the place of personal effort.

Sons and Daughters of God, 263.

AS A people, we are not deficient in talent. There are men and women among us whose labors God would accept if they would offer them to Him, but there are so very few who have the spirit of sacrifice. Some will hand out readily of their means, and feel that when they have done this, there is no more required of them. They make no special sacrifice in thus doing. Money is good as far as it goes, but, unless accompanied by personal effort, will go but a little way toward converting souls to the truth. Not only does God call for your money, . . . but He calls for you. While you have given of your means, you have selfishly withheld yourselves. One earnest worker in the vineyard is worth more than a million of money without men to do the work. This giving of yourselves will be a sacrifice if you have a correct estimate of the work, and realize its claims.

359. Christ will work with those who give not only of their means, but also of themselves in relieving some of His afflicted ones.

Spalding and Magan, 140.

I WAS in prison, and ye came unto me." We shall have to give of our means to support laborers in the harvest field, and we shall rejoice in the sheaves gathered in. But while this is right, there is a work as yet untouched that must be done. The mission of Christ was to heal the sick, encourage the hopeless, bind up the brokenhearted. This work of restoration is to be carried on among the needy suffering ones of humanity. God calls not only for your benevolence, but your cheerful countenance, your hopeful works, the grasp of your hand. Relieve some of God's afflicted ones. Some are sick and hope has departed. Bring back the sunlight to them. There are souls who have lost their courage; speak to them, pray for them. There are those who need the bread of life. Read to them from the Word of God. There is a soul sickness no balm can reach, no medicine heal. Pray for them, and bring them to Jesus Christ. And in all your work, Christ will be present to make impressions upon the human hearts.

360. Every one of us is to be a Christian philanthropist in doing medical missionary work.

Review and Herald, vol. 6, 441.

INTELLIGENT, self-denying, self-sacrificing men are now needed, men who realize the solemnity and importance of God's work, and who as Christian philanthropists will fulfill the commission of Christ. The medical missionary work given us to do means something to every one of us. It is a work of soul saving; it is the proclamation of the gospel message.

361. True medical missionaries will carry in one hand relief for the sin-sick and in the other hand relief for the physically sick.

Medical Ministry, 328.

IN ONE hand they are to carry the gospel for the relief of sin-burdened souls; and in the other hand they are to carry remedies for the relief of physical suffering. Thus they will be true medical missionaries for God.

362. Christ will come near to instruct us in practical lessons of how to care for suffering humanity.

Pacific Union Recorder, 2.

ALL can labor for the salvation of those who are out of the ark of safety. When church members stand pledged to the service of God, pledged to do missionary work; when they take hold of the work unselfishly, because they love the souls for whom Christ died, and are desirous of uniting with the Great Missionary, He will come very near to them to instruct them. Life is full of opportunities for the practical missionary. Every man, woman, and child can sow each day the seeds of kind words and unselfish deeds. The world is not a playground where we are to amuse ourselves; it is a school in which we are to study earnestly and thoroughly the lessons given in the Word of God. There we may learn how to receive and how to impart. There we may learn how to seek for souls in the highways and byways of life. If those who engage so earnestly in the games of this world would strive as earnestly for the crown of life which fadeth not away, what victories they would gain! They would become true missionaries, and would see how much could be done to relieve suffering humanity. What a blessing this would be! What we need is practical education. When ministers and people practice the lessons Christ has given in His Word, they will become Christlike in character.

363. A breath of life will come into our churches when they combine medical missionary work with the proclamation of the third angel's message.

Loma Linda Messages, 74.

COMBINE medical missionary work with the proclamation of the third angel's message. Make regular, organized efforts to lift the churches out of the dead level in which they have been for years. Send out into the churches workers who will set the principles of health reform before every church in Michigan. See if the breath of life will not then come into these churches.

364. We are to train and work quickly, to prevent the enemy from possessing the fields now open before us.

The Lord's Work

Loma Linda Messages, 58.

WORKERS—gospel medical missionaries—are needed now. We cannot afford to spend years in preparation. Soon doors now open to the truth will be forever closed. Carry the message now. Do not wait, allowing the enemy to take possession of fields now open before you. Let little companies go forth to do the work to which Christ appointed His disciples. Let them labor as evangelists, scattering our publications, and talking of the truth to those they meet. Let them pray for the sick, ministering to their necessities not with drugs, but with nature's remedies, and teaching them how to regain health and avoid disease.

365. There are those who can do acceptable medical missionary work with only a few months of instruction.

The Paulson Collection, 38.

THERE are those who with a few months' instruction would be prepared to go out and do acceptable medical missionary work. Some cannot feel that it is their duty to give years to one line of study.

366. If we are doing our best to relieve suffering, God will give us knowledge from the higher school.

Special Testimonies, Series B, 214–215.

MANY will go out to labor for the Master who have not been able to take a regular course of study in school. God will help those workers. They will obtain knowledge from the higher school, and will be fitted to take their position in the rank and file of workers as nurses. The great Medical Missionary sees every effort that is made to find access to souls by presenting the principles of health reform.

Decided changes are taking place in our world. The Lord has declared that He will turn and overturn. Humble men, who hitherto have been in obscurity, must now be given opportunity to become workers.

To those who go out to do medical missionary work, I would say, Serve the Lord Jesus Christ with sanctified understanding, in connection with the ministers of the gospel and the great Teacher. He who has given you your commission will give you skill and understanding as you consecrate yourselves to His service, engaging diligently in labor and study, doing your best to bring relief to the sick and suffering.

367. All can become intelligent in health matters by studying our literature.

Medical Ministry, 320.

BUT few can take a course of training in our medical institutions. But all can study our health literature, and become intelligent on this important subject.

368. We need to appreciate and study more the books written for our instruction in medical missionary work.

Testimonies, vol. 7, 63.

LET our people show that they have a living interest in medical missionary work. Let them prepare themselves for usefulness by studying the books that have been written for our instruction in these lines. These books deserve much more attention and appreciation than they have received.

369. Heaven's plan is that we use the simple, economical agencies of nature in our health work.

Testimonies, vol. 5, 443.

THERE are many ways of practicing the healing art, but there is only one way that Heaven approves. God's remedies are the simple agencies of nature that will not tax or debilitate the system through their powerful properties. Pure air and water, cleanliness, a proper diet, purity of life, and a firm trust in God are remedies for the want of which thousands are dying; yet these remedies are going out of date because their skillful use requires work that the people do not appreciate. Fresh air, exercise, pure water, and clean, sweet premises are within the reach of all with but little expense.

370. Every person is to be knowledgeable in the application of the eight true remedies.

The Ministry of Healing, 127.

PURE air, sunlight, abstemiousness, rest, exercise, proper diet, the use of water, trust in divine power these are the true remedies. Every person should have a knowledge of nature's remedial agencies and how to apply them.

371. The explanation of natural law and the urgency of obedience to it is part of the third angel's message.

Counsels on Health, 21.

TO MAKE natural law plain, and to urge obedience to it, is a work that accompanies the third angel's message. Ignorance is no excuse now for the transgression of law.

372. To follow in the footsteps of Jesus, we must help the sick as He did.

My Life Today, 227.

JESUS came in personal contact with men. He did not stand aloof and apart from those who needed His help. He entered the homes of men, comforted the mourner, healed the sick, aroused the careless, and went about doing good. And if we follow in the footsteps of Jesus, we must do as He did. We must give men the same kind of help that He did.

373. We must relieve physical necessities as did Christ if we are to reach the hearts of our fellow men.

Testimonies, vol. 9, 127.

CHRIST'S example must be followed by those who claim to be His children. Relieve the physical necessities of your fellow men, and their gratitude will break down the barriers, and enable you to reach their hearts.

374. We are not to delay in the medical missionary work Christ has commissioned us to do for Him.

Loma Linda Messages, 384.

CHRIST is no longer in this world in person, to go through our cities and towns and villages, healing the sick. He has commissioned us to carry forward the medical missionary work that He began; and in this work we are to do our very best. . . . I have been instructed that we are not to delay to do the work that needs to be done in health reform lines.

375. The heavenly messengers will soon pass by those who delay in doing what they can.

Loma Linda Messages, 83.

THERE will soon be an awakening that will surprise many. Those who do not realize the necessity of what is to be done, will be passed by, and the heavenly messengers will work with those who are called the common people, fitting them to carry the truth to many places. Now is the time for us to awake and do what we can.

376. Christ will raise up and instruct those who are willing to do His will.

Testimonies, vol. 7, 101–102.

I WILL instruct the ignorant, and anoint with heavenly eyesalve the eyes of many who are now in spiritual darkness. I will raise up agents who will carry out My will to prepare a people to stand before Me in the time of the end.

377. We will see thousands of streams of medical missionary work cover the earth.

Medical Ministry, 317.

WE SHALL see the medical missionary work broadening and deepening at every point of its progress, because of the inflowing of hundreds and thousands of streams, until the whole earth is covered as the waters cover the sea.

378. Our first work is to study in agricultural lines, the A, B, and C of education.

Testimonies, vol. 6, 179.

STUDY in agricultural lines should be the A, B, and C of the education given in our schools. This is the very first work that should be entered upon.

379. It is highly important that the study of physiology occupy first place in the studies of childhood.

Healthful Living, 484.

A PRACTICAL knowledge of the science of human life is necessary in order to glorify God in our bodies. It is therefore of the highest importance that among studies selected for childhood, physiology should occupy the first place.

It is well that physiology is introduced into the common schools as a branch of education. All children should study it. It should be regarded as the basis of all educational effort.

380. Obedience to natural law is the condition for success in agriculture.

Child Guidance, 56.

NO ONE can succeed in agriculture or gardening without attention to the laws involved. The special needs of every variety of plant must be studied. Different varieties require different soil and cultivation, and compliance with the laws governing each is the condition of success. . . . In cultivating carefulness, patience, attention to detail, obedience to law, it imparts a most essential training.

381. Obedience to the divine laws of nature is the only way to recover or preserve health.

Loma Linda Messages, 110.

THE laws of nature, as truly as the precepts of the Decalogue, are divine, and only in obedience to them can health be recovered or preserved.

382. God ordained modern inventions to lighten the labor in cultivating the soil.

The Seventh-day Adventist Bible Commentary, vol. 1, 1089.

THE greater the length of time the earth has lain under the curse, the more difficult has it been for man to cultivate it, and make it productive. As the soil has become more barren, and double labor has had to be expended upon it, God has raised up men with inventive faculties to construct implements to lighten labor on the land groaning under the curse.

383. The development of rapid transportation is an example of God using even unrepentant man to carry out His will.

Fundamentals of Christian Education, 409.

THE knowledge current in the world may be acquired; for all men are God's property, and are worked by God to fulfill His will in certain lines, even when they refuse the man Christ Jesus as their Saviour. The way in which God uses men is not always discerned, but He does use them. God entrusts men with talents and inventive genius, in order that His great work in our world may be accomplished. The inventions of human minds are supposed to spring from humanity, but God is behind all. He has caused that the means of rapid traveling shall have been invented, for the great day of His preparation.

384. The great Physician cooperates with everyone who works to relieve suffering humanity.

Spalding and Magan, 127.

THE great Physician cooperates with every effort made in the behalf of suffering humanity. . . . His heart of sympathy goes out to all earth's sufferers, and with every one who works for their relief He cooperates.

385. Disobedience to the laws of health makes the use of drugs a necessity.

Medical Ministry, 222.

THE disuse of meats, with healthful dishes nicely prepared to take the place of flesh meats, would place a large number of the sick and suffering ones in a fair way of recovering their health, without the use of drugs. But if the physician encourages a meat-eating diet to his invalid patients, then he will make a necessity for the use of drugs.

386. Those who persist in the use of unhealthful substances will feel the need of drugs.

Counsels on Health, 261.

EDUCATE away from drugs. Use them less and less, and depend more upon hygienic agencies; then nature will respond to God's physicians, pure air, pure water, proper exercise, a clear conscience. Those who persist in the use of tea, coffee, and flesh meats will feel the need of drugs, but many might recover without one grain of medicine, if they would live out the laws of health. Drugs need seldom be used.

387. Our physicians should almost entirely dispense with medicine.

Pamphlet 66, Health, Philanthropic, and Medical Missionary Work, 40.

SHOULD our physicians who claim to believe the truth almost entirely dispense with medicine, and faithfully practice along the lines of the principles of hygiene, using nature's remedies, far greater success would attend their efforts.

388. Those who are benefactors of the race are reflecting the rays of the Sun of Righteousness.

The Desire of Ages, 464–465.

THE world has had its great teachers, men of giant intellect and wonderful research, men whose utterances have stimulated thought, and opened to view vast fields of knowledge; and these men have been honored as guides and benefactors of their race. . . . As the moon and stars of the solar system shine by the reflected light of the sun, so, as far as their teaching is true, do the world's great thinkers reflect the rays of the Sun of Righteousness. Every gem of thought, every flash of the intellect, is from the Light of the world.

389. Every impulse of love to bless and uplift others is the working of the Holy Spirit.

Christ's Object Lessons, 385.

WHEREVER there is an impulse of love and sympathy, wherever the heart reaches out to bless and uplift others, there is revealed the working of God's Holy Spirit. . . . [Such] acts show the working of a divine power.

390. God works by His own natural laws.

Manuscript Releases, vol. 15, 220.

THE sequence of nature is under God's jurisdiction. God works by His own laws, for He is a God of order.

391. Natural law operates in a predictable, consistent manner.

Christ's Object Lessons, 84.

IN THE laws of God in nature, effect follows cause with unerring certainty.

392. The rapid increase in scientific knowledge is ordained of God.

Patriarchs and Prophets, 113.

GOD has permitted a flood of light to be poured upon the world in both science and art.

393. Cooperation with the Creator is the only way to success in temporal as well as spiritual lines.

Christ's Object Lessons, 82.

WHENEVER man accomplishes anything, whether in spiritual or in temporal lines, he should bear in mind that he does it through cooperation with his Maker.

394. Through some modern inventions Satan leads man to forget God.

The Seventh-day Adventist Bible Commentary, vol. 1, 1089.

BUT God has not been in all man's inventions. Satan has controlled the minds of men to a great extent, and has hurried men to new inventions which has led them to forget God.

395. The Lord has pointed out the work of Seventh-day Adventists, which is distinct from that which the Lord has ordained for the Salvation Army.

Testimonies, vol. 8, 184–185.

THE Lord has marked out our way of working. As a people we are not to imitate and fall in with Salvation Army methods. This is not the work that the Lord has given us to do. Neither is it our work to condemn them and speak harsh words against them. There are precious, self-sacrificing souls in the Salvation Army. We are to treat them kindly. There are in the Army honest souls, who are sincerely serving the Lord and who will see greater light, advancing to the acceptance of all truth. The Salvation Army workers are trying to save the neglected, downtrodden ones. Discourage them not. Let them do that class of work by their own methods and in their own way. But the Lord has plainly pointed out the work that Seventh-day Adventists are to do.

396. God's work for His people is not to be interfered with by supporting good tasks that have not been assigned to them.

Testimonies, vol. 6, 286.

TO CARE for these needy ones is a good work; yet in this age of the world the Lord does not give us as a people directions to establish large and expensive institutions for this purpose. If, however, there are among us individuals who feel called of God to establish institutions for the care of orphan children, let them follow out their convictions of duty. But in caring for the world's poor they should appeal to the world for support. They are not to draw upon the people to whom the Lord has given the most important work ever given to men, the work of bringing the last message of mercy before all nations, kindreds, tongues, and people. The Lord's treasury must have a surplus to sustain the work of the gospel in "regions beyond."

397. We are to always study and teach the simplest remedies accessible to the common people.

Selected Messages, book 2, 298–299.

ALWAYS study and teach the use of the simplest remedies, and the special blessing of the Lord may be expected to follow the use of these means which are within the reach of the common people.

398. The advancement of the work of God does not require costly buildings, furnishings, or equipment.

The Ministry of Healing, 36.

WEALTH or high position, costly equipment, architecture or furnishings, are not essential to the advancement of the work of God.

399. Many costly inventions are not needed in God's simple plan for education.

Loma Linda Messages, 355.

THERE are many inventions which cost large sums of money which it is just as well should not come into our work. They are not what our students need. Let the education given be simple in its nature.

400. We need to emphasize those methods and technologies that the patients can utilize at home.

Spalding and Magan, 390.

THOSE who go from the Sanitarium should go so well instructed that they can teach others the methods of treating their families. There is danger of spending far too much money on machinery and appliances which the patients can never use in their home lessons.

401. We are to move slowly in the acquisition of equipment which requires experts to operate.

Loma Linda Messages, 178.

NOW I am certain that great care should be taken in purchasing electrical instruments and costly mechanical fixtures. Move slowly, Brother Burden, and do not trust to men who suppose that they understand what is essential, and who launch out in spending money for many things that require experts to handle them.

402. We are to make prominent those principles that will live through the eternal ages.

Lift Him Up, 366.

GOD has given man immortal principles to which every human power must one day bow. He has given us truth in trust. The precious beams of this light are not to be hidden under a bushel, but are to give light to all that are in the house. Truth, imperishable truth is to be made prominent. Show those with whom you come in contact that the truth is of consequence to you. It means much to you to stand by the principles that will live through the eternal ages.

403. All conflict with natural law creates a diseased soul.

The Health Reformer, 215.

EVERYTHING that conflicts with natural law creates a diseased condition of the soul.

404. We need to avoid praiseworthy work that has not been placed in our hands by the Lord.

Spalding and Magan, 116.

THERE is always a danger of taking upon ourselves a work the Lord has not placed in our hands, and neglecting that which He has given us to do, and which would better honor His name; that which to human eyes may appear praiseworthy, may be the very thing the Lord has not placed in our hands.

405. God expects us to destroy the destructive and health-threatening vermin.

Selected Messages, book 3, 329.

THIS earth has been cursed because of sin, and in these last days vermin of every kind will multiply. These pests must be killed, or they will annoy and torment and even kill us, and destroy the work of our hands and the fruit of our land. In places there are ants [termites] which entirely destroy the woodwork of houses. Should not these be destroyed? Fruit trees must be sprayed, that the insects which would spoil the fruit may be killed. God has given us a part to act, and this part we must act with faithfulness. Then we can leave the rest with the Lord.

406. We are to place ourselves in the condition most favorable to the recovery of health.

Spalding and Magan, 7.

I THANK the Lord that it is our privilege to cooperate with Him in the work of restoration, availing ourselves of all possible advantages in the recovery of health. It is no denial of our faith to place ourselves in the condition most favorable to recovery.

407. At times we have to be guided by the concept of the benefit outweighing the potential harm.

Testimonies, vol. 2, 373.

WHEN I have been from home sometimes, I have known that the bread upon the table, and the food generally, would hurt me; but I would be obliged to eat a little to sustain life.

408. It is God's will that we use as needed every facility for the restoration of health that is in harmony with natural law.

The Ministry of Healing, 231–232.

IT IS not a denial of faith to use such remedies as God has provided to alleviate pain and to aid nature in her work of restoration. It is no denial of faith to cooperate with God, and to place themselves in the condition most favorable to recovery. God has put it in our power to obtain a knowledge of the laws of life. This knowledge has been placed within our reach for use. We should employ every facility for the restoration of health, taking every advantage possible, working in harmony with natural laws.

409. All true recovery from disease is from God.

The Ministry of Healing, 113.

ALL life-giving power is from Him. When one recovers from disease, it is God who restores him.

410. Strong coffee may be used as a medicine, but coffee is not to be used as a beverage.

Selected Messages, book 2, 302–303.

I HAVE not knowingly drunk a cup of genuine coffee for twenty years, only, as I stated, during my sickness for a medicine I drank a cup of coffee, very strong, with a raw egg broken into it.

411. Tea also may be used as a medicine, but not as a beverage.

Selected Messages, book 2, 302.

I DO not use tea, either green or black. Not a spoonful has passed my lips for many years except when crossing the ocean, and once since on this side I took it as a medicine when I was sick and vomiting. In such circumstances it may prove a present relief.

412. Ellen G. White received X-ray treatments, for which she was grateful.

Selected Messages, book 2, 303.

FOR several weeks I took treatment with the X-ray for the black spot that was on my forehead. In all I took twenty-three treatments, and these succeeded in entirely removing the mark. For this I am very grateful.

413. Blood transfusions are suggested as a means of saving lives.

Medical Ministry, 286–287.

THERE is one thing that has saved life an infusion of blood from one person to another; but this would be difficult and perhaps impossible for you to do. I merely suggest it.

414. Our prophetess received and recommended receiving the smallpox vaccine.

Selected Messages, book 2, 303.

YOU ask for definite and concise information regarding what Sister White wrote about vaccination and serum.

This question can be answered very briefly for so far as we have any record, she did not refer to them in any of her writings.

You will be interested to know, however, that at a time when there was an epidemic of smallpox in the vicinity, she herself was vaccinated and urged her helpers, those connected with her, to be vaccinated. In taking this step Sister White recognized the fact that it has been proven that vaccination either renders one immune from smallpox or greatly lightens its effects if one does come down with it. She also recognized the danger of exposing others if they failed to take this precaution. D. E. Robinson, E. G. White secretary.

415. Needed surgical operations are to be undertaken.

Selected Messages, book 2, 284–285.

IT IS our privilege to use every God-appointed means in correspondence with our faith, and then trust in God, when we have urged the promise. If there is need of a surgical operation, and the physician is willing to undertake the case, it is not a denial of faith to have the operation performed. After the patient has committed his will to the will of God, let him trust, drawing nigh to the Great Physician, the Mighty Healer, and giving himself up in perfect trust. The Lord will honor his faith in the very manner He sees is for His own name's glory.

416. Scientific health institutions are ordained of God even though He will work powerfully through those untrained by them.

Testimonies, vol. 5, 82.

GOD will work a work in our day that but few anticipate. He will raise up and exalt among us those who are taught rather by the unction of His Spirit than by the outward training of scientific institutions. These facilities are not to be despised or condemned; they are ordained of God, but they can furnish only the exterior qualifications. God will manifest that He is not dependent on learned, self-important mortals.

417. We need to place confidence in those whom we choose to care for us.

Testimonies, vol. 3, 78–79.

WHILE you fear to trust yourself in the hands of the physicians, and think that you understand your case better than they do, you cannot be benefited, but only harmed, by their treatment of your case. Unless physicians can obtain the confidence of their patients, they can never help them. If you prescribe for yourself, and think you know what treatment you should have, better than the physicians do, you cannot be benefited. You must yield your will and ideas, and not rein yourself up to resist their judgment and advice in your case.

418. Strong stimulants and all the restorative means readily available were utilized in the attempt to prevent the death of Elder James White.

A Sketch of the Last Sickness and Death of Elder James White, (a statement by Dr. J. H. Kellogg),19–20.

AT 8 P.M. (Aug.5, 1881) I examined his pulse, and remarked the same peculiarity observed the previous evening, weakness and unusual frequency, although there was no fever, neither any evidence of chill, the body being warm. He expressed himself as feeling entirely comfortable, but inclined to sleep. About five minutes later I examined his pulse again, and observed a slight irregularity. Strong stimulants were immediately administered, and Mrs. White and a number of special friends were advised that his condition was critical.

The grave symptoms grew rapidly worse for an hour, notwithstanding the most vigorous efforts which could be made by the use of stimulating and restorative means of every sort, which were ready at hand. . . .

At 10 A. M. (Aug.6, 1881)he was able to converse a little in brief sentences, but his pupils were still dilated and the symptoms of paralysis of certain portions of the brain, which had appeared in the night, continued.

With the concurrence of the friends, we called in consultation Dr. Millspaugh of the city, whom we found in entire agreement with us in reference to the condition and the appropriate treatment.

About 1 P. M. his pulse suddenly began to increase in frequency, and soon became very feeble and irregular. Within thirty minutes he became unconscious, and his pulse rapidly rose to 176, and his respiration to 60 per minute. His temperature was 99 degrees, one-half degree above the normal temperature. The same measures used with the previous attack were again employed, but without effect, and he remained in the condition described until he breathed his last, just after 5 P. M.

419. When in danger of death we are to do the best we can, even to the giving of quinine for malaria.

Selected Messages, book 2, 281–282.

ONE time while we were in Australia, a brother who had been acting as a missionary in the islands, told mother of the sickness and death of his first-born son. He was seriously afflicted with malaria, and his father was advised to give him quinine, but in view of the counsel in the Testimonies to avoid the use of quinine he refused to administer it, and his son died. When he met Sister White, he asked her this question: "Would I have sinned to give the boy quinine when I knew of no other way to check malaria and when the prospect was that he would die without it?" In reply she said, "No, we are expected to do the best we can." W. C. White Letter, Sept.10, 1935.

420. Our medical personnel are not to honor any one system of health-care, but are to know the very best from many systems.

The Medical Evangelist, October/November, 1911, 132, (as quoted in *A Compendium on Outpost Evangelism*, by James and David Lee, Fourth Edition, 1986, 540).

WHEN questioned regarding the work to be done at Loma Linda, Mrs. White said during the Mountain View Conference in January 1910, Whatever our young people, preparing to be physicians need to know, that we must prepare to teach.

Our medical missionaries should be given the opportunities to know the very best things done by the allopaths, the eclectics, the homeopaths, the osteopaths, [the "naturopaths"] and the water-cure doctors, but none of these systems should be adopted as comprising that which our physicians need to know: nor should the name of any of these systems be adopted as the "sign of our order." Neither should our medical men give the credit or honor of the results of their labors under God, to any man or group of men, or to any locality, or to any system.

421. Dr. Kellogg used the Spirit of Prophecy as a guide in determining truth in the area of medical knowledge.

How Kellogg Kept Ahead, E. G. White Publication Document File 45, Windows, 144.

HE [Doctor Kellogg] said when a new thing is brought out in the medical world he knew from his knowledge of the Spirit of Prophecy whether it belonged in our system or not. If it did, he instantly adopted it and advertised it while the rest of the doctors were slowly feeling their way, and when they finally adopted it, he had five years the start of them.

On the other hand when the medical profession were swept off their feet by some new fad, if it did not fit the light we had received [from Ellen White] he simply did not touch it. When the doctors finally discovered their mistake, they wondered how it came that Dr. Kellogg did not get caught.

422. In spite of using all the means that they could, Ellen White's fourth son died in infancy of erysipelas.

Testimonies, vol. 1, 245.

THE next morning he (Ellen White's infant fourth son John Herbert) was taken very sick. It was an extreme case of erysipelas in the face and head. . . . My dear babe was a great sufferer. Twenty-four days and nights we anxiously watched over him, using all the means that we could for his recovery and earnestly presenting his case to the Lord. . . . But our heavenly Father saw fit to remove the loved one.

423. The White's oldest son died at the age of sixteen years from pneumonia.

The Health Reformer, 122.

MY MIND goes back to Oak Hill Cemetery in Battle Creek, Michigan. I see there two graves. My noble first-born son (Henry) fills the long grave. Next comes a short grave where lies my darling babe, my last-born. The first died (Dec. 8, 1863) of inflammation of the lungs after a sickness of eight days. . . . The second died (Dec. 14, 1860) from sleeping in a room that had not been used for two weeks.

424. Although the earth is waxing old like a garment, God will never cease to bless the cultivation of the soil.

Testimonies, vol. 6, 178.

IF THE land is cultivated, it will, with the blessing of God, supply our necessities. We are not to be discouraged about temporal things because of apparent failures, nor should we be disheartened by delay. We should work the soil cheerfully, hopefully, gratefully, believing that the earth holds in her bosom rich stores for the faithful worker to garner, stores richer than gold or silver. The niggardliness laid to her charge is false witness. With proper, intelligent cultivation the earth will yield its treasures for the benefit of man. The mountains and hills are changing; the earth is waxing old like a garment; but the blessing of God, which spreads a table for His people in the wilderness, will never cease.

425. Angels will cause the earth to yield its gardening treasures.

Spalding Magan Unpublished Testimonies, 446–447.

YOU are to prepare the ground for the sowing of the seed; and in your efforts the blessing of the Lord will certainly be with you if you will walk humbly with God. . . .

You are not working alone. When you are tempted to become discouraged remember this. Angels of God are right around you. They will minister to the very earth, causing it to give forth its treasures.

426. Ninety percent of the sick will recover if they perseveringly live out the principles of health reform.

Medical Ministry, 224.

IF THE sick and suffering will do only as well as they know in regard to living out the principles of health reform perseveringly, then they will in nine cases out of ten recover from their ailments.

427. Sickness will be rare in those who intelligently regard their bodily necessities.

Selected Messages, book 2, 291.

BUT if all would seek to become intelligent in regard to their bodily necessities, sickness would be rare instead of common. An ounce of prevention is worth a pound of cure.

428. It is urgent that we move into the country, where we can raise our own produce.

Christian Leadership, 21.

WHEN power is allied with wickedness, it is allied to satanic agencies, and it will work to destroy those who are the Lord's property. . . . For this reason I see the necessity of the people of God moving out of the cities into retired country [places,] where they may cultivate the land and raise their own produce. Thus they may bring their children up with simple, healthful habits. I see the necessity of making haste to get all things ready for the crisis.

429. We have but a moment of respite in which to do the work assigned us by the Lord.

Maranatha, 266.

A MOMENT of respite has been graciously given us of God. Every power lent us of heaven is to be used in doing the work assigned us by the Lord for those who are perishing in ignorance. The warning message is to be sounded in all parts of the world. . . . A great work is to be done, and this work has been entrusted to those who know the truth for this time.

The Final Work

430. The work we have neglected to do will have to be done during crisis times.

Testimonies, vol. 5, 463.

THE work which the church has failed to do in a time of peace and prosperity she will have to do in a terrible crisis under most discouraging, forbidding circumstances. The warnings that worldly conformity has silenced or withheld must be given under the fiercest opposition from enemies of the faith.

431. As the Spirit of God withdraws from the earth, the movements will be rapid ones.

Testimonies, vol. 9, 11.

WE ARE living in the time of the end. The fast-fulfilling signs of the times declare that the coming of Christ is near at hand. The days in which we live are solemn and important. The Spirit of God is gradually but surely being withdrawn from the earth. Plagues and judgments are already falling upon the despisers of the grace of God. The calamities by land and sea, the unsettled state of society, the alarms of war, are portentous. They forecast approaching events of the greatest magnitude. The agencies of evil are combining their forces and consolidating. They are strengthening for the last great crisis. Great changes are soon to take place in our world, and the final movements will be rapid ones.

432. God's people will do a quick, triumphant work.

Battle Creek Letters, 49–50.

MY PEOPLE are to do a sharp quick work. Those who with purity of purpose fully consecrate themselves to Me, body, mind, and spirit, shall work in My way and in My name.

Battle Creek Letters, 57.

THE kingdoms of this world are soon to become the kingdoms of our Lord and of his Christ. . . . There is to be a rapid and triumphant spread of the gospel.

433. Though more difficult than previously, the Lord's work will be done.

The Paulson Collection, 109.

THAT which should have been done twenty, yea, more than twenty years ago, is now to be done speedily. The work will be more difficult to do now than it would have been years ago, but it will be done.

434. Soon ministers will be able to minister only on the gospel plan of ministering—medical missionary work.

Counsels on Health, 533.

I WISH to tell you that soon there will be no work done in ministerial lines but medical missionary work. The work of a minister is to minister. Our ministers are to work on the gospel plan of ministering. . . . You will never be ministers after the gospel order till you show a decided interest in medical missionary work, the gospel of healing and blessing and strengthening.

435. Every soul that will work under Christ's directions will be enlisted in the struggle against Satan's army.

Testimonies, vol. 6, 237.

CHRIST says: "Where Satan has set his throne, there shall stand My cross. Satan shall be cast out, and I will be lifted up to draw all men unto Me. I will become the center of the redeemed world. The Lord God shall be exalted. Those who are now controlled by human ambition, human passions, shall become workers for Me. Evil influences have conspired to counterwork all good. They have confederated to make men think it righteous to oppose the law of Jehovah. But My army shall meet in conflict with the satanic force. My Spirit shall combine with every heavenly agency to oppose them. I will engage every sanctified human agency in the universe. None of My agencies are to be absent. I have work for all who love Me, employment for every soul who will work under My direction. The activity of Satan's army, the danger that surrounds the human soul, calls for the energies of every worker."

436. There will be plenty of suffering ones in need of intelligent care in the perilous times before us.

Counsels on Health, 504, 506.

PERILOUS times are before us. The whole world will be involved in perplexity and distress, disease of every kind will be upon the human family, and such ignorance as now prevails concerning the laws of health would result in great suffering and the loss of many lives that might be saved. . . .

As religious aggression subverts the liberties of our nation, those who would stand for freedom of conscience will be placed in unfavorable positions. For their own sake, they should, while they have opportunity, become intelligent in regard to disease, its causes, prevention, and cure. And those who do this will find a field of labor anywhere. There will be suffering ones, plenty of them, who will need help, not only among those of our own faith, but largely among those who know not the truth.

437. Obedience to God's physical, mental, and moral laws is a prerequisite to being restored to His harmonious universe.

Education, 99–100.

THE laws that govern the heart's action, regulating the flow of the current of life to the body, are the laws of the mighty Intelligence that has the jurisdiction of the soul. From Him all life proceeds. Only in harmony with Him can be found its true sphere of action. For all the objects of His creation the condition is the same a life sustained by receiving the life of God, a life exercised in harmony with the Creator's will. To transgress His law, physical, mental, or moral, is to place one's self out of harmony with the universe, to introduce discord, anarchy, ruin.

438. The transgression of natural as well as spiritual laws must be confessed and forsaken.

The Ministry of Healing, 228.

IT SHOULD be made plain that the violation of God's law, either natural or spiritual, is sin, and that in order . . . to receive His blessings, sin must be confessed and forsaken.

439. In order to understand the Bible and the object of life, we must know our physical organism, and we must care for it aright.

The Health Reformer, 45.

CHRISTIANS, above all others, should be awake to this important subject, and should become intelligent in regard to their own organism. Says the psalmist, "I will praise thee, for I am fearfully and wonderfully made." If we would be able to comprehend the truths of God's Word, and the object and purpose of our living, we must know ourselves, and understand how to relate our selves rightly to life and to health.

440. We are to carefully study every mechanism of our physical being.

My Life Today, 127.

THIS living machinery is to be understood. Every part of its wonderful mechanism is to be carefully studied.

441. Health education is to be a part of the work of every gospel worker.

Review and Herald, vol. 6, 244.

EVERY gospel worker should feel that the giving of instruction in the principles of healthful living is a part of his appointed work.

442. School teachers are to be intelligent in regard to disease, its causes, and the importance of the laws of life.

Australasian Record, 277.

THOSE who act as teachers are to be intelligent in regard to disease and its causes, understanding that every action of the human agent should be in perfect harmony with the laws of life.

443. A knowledge of how to treat the sick will make us welcome any place.

Healthful Living, 272.

THEY need an education in the science of how to treat the sick, for this will give them a welcome in any place.

444. Genuine medical missionaries will know how to teach the principles of healthful living and also how to give the simple treatments for the sick.

My Life Today, 226.

GOD'S people are to be genuine medical missionaries. They are to learn to minister to the needs of soul and body. They should know how to give the simple treatments that do so much to relieve pain and remove disease. They should be familiar with the principles of health reform, that they may show others how, by right habits of eating, drinking, and dressing, disease may be prevented and health regained.

445. We are to teach the sick that the most effective remedies are the natural remedies God has provided.

Medical Ministry, 225.

THE sick should be educated to have confidence in nature's great blessings which God has provided; and the most effective remedies for disease are pure soft water, the blessed God-given sunshine coming into the rooms of the invalids, living outdoors as much as possible, having healthful exercise, eating and drinking foods that are prepared in the most healthful manner.

446. The intelligent use of the God given roots and herbs will decrease the frequency with which a physician is needed.

Medical Ministry, 230–231.

GOD has caused to grow out of the ground herbs for the use of man, and if we understand the nature of these roots and herbs, and make a right use of them, there would not be a necessity of running for the doctor so frequently, and people would be in much better health than they are today.

447. Some simple herbs can be used to prevent and treat disease.

Selected Messages, book 2, 294.

THE Lord has given some simple herbs of the field that at times are beneficial; and if every family were educated in how to use these herbs in case of sickness, much suffering might be prevented, and no doctor need be called. These old-fashioned, simple herbs, used intelligently, would have recovered many sick.

448. Charcoal can be beneficial when there is inflammation caused by infection, even if associated with bruising.

Selected Messages, book 2, 294.

ONE of the most beneficial remedies is pulverized charcoal, placed in a bag and used in fomentations. This is a most successful remedy. . . . To students when injured with bruised hands and suffering with inflammation, I have prescribed this simple remedy, with perfect success. . . . The most severe inflammation of the eyes will be relieved by a poultice of charcoal, put in a bag, and dipped in hot or cold water, as will best suit the case. This works like a charm.

449. We are to treat the sick with God's natural remedies and teach them to have faith in His healing power.

The Desire of Ages, 824–825.

FOR the sick we should use the remedies which God has provided in nature, and we should point them to Him who alone can restore. It is our work to present the sick and suffering to Christ in the arms of our faith. We should teach them to believe in the Great Healer. We should lay hold on His promise, and pray for the manifestation of His power. The very essence of the gospel is restoration, and the Saviour would have us bid the sick, the hopeless, and the afflicted take hold upon His strength.

450. When we are sick, we are to have the health workers do all that they can in our behalf, while we look to Christ our Sin bearer.

Manuscript Releases, vol. 7, 376.

LET those who are sick have hope and courage to bring their cases to the Master. The angels of God are here. While the physicians and the helpers are doing everything they can on your behalf, Christ Himself is the Healer of your diseases. He it is who combats the disease you have brought on yourself by an imprudent, sinful course of action. He, the Sin-bearer, is the only One who can successfully combat disease. Oh, link up with the Great Physician! He is ready to place His everlasting arms underneath you.

451. When praying for healing, one must confess and forsake disobedience to God's natural and spiritual laws.

The Ministry of Healing, 228.

TO THOSE who desire prayer for their restoration to health, it should be made plain that the violation of God's law, either natural or spiritual, is sin, and that in order for them to receive His blessing, sin must be confessed and forsaken.

452. God does not heal us when we refuse to utilize the means of healing that lie within our reach.

The Paulson Collection, 26.

GOD does not heal the sick without the aid of the means of healing which lie within the reach of man; or when men refuse to be benefited by the simple remedies that God has provided in pure air and water.

453. Unless we are using God's simple, readily available remedies, there is no use to pray for healing.

The Paulson Collection, 48.

IT IS of no use to have seasons of prayer for the sick, while they refuse to use the simple remedies which God has provided, and which are close by them.

454. When we pray for a miracle, God directs us to the simple remedies through which He will often work to restore the sick.

The Seventh-day Adventist Bible Commentary, vol. 7, 938.

GOD'S miracles do not always bear the outward semblance of miracles. Often they are brought about in a way which looks like the natural course of events. When we pray for the sick, we also work for them. We answer our own prayers by using the remedies within our reach. . . .

Natural means, used in accordance with God's will, bring about supernatural results. We ask for a miracle, and the Lord directs the mind to some simple remedy.

455. Success in treating the sick will follow the reformation of health habits, the use of nature's remedies, and trust in divine power.

Review and Herald, vol. 6, 319.

THE true medical missionary will be wise in the treatment of the sick, using the remedies that nature provides. And then he will look to Christ as the true healer of diseases. The principles of health reform brought into the life of the patient, the use of nature's remedies, and the co-operation of divine agencies in behalf of the suffering, will bring success.

456. We are to first use the agencies that God has provided, then we are to ask for His blessing.

The Paulson Collection, 29–30.

I BELIEVE in calling upon the Great Physician when we have used the remedies I have mentioned. . . . We cannot heal. We cannot change the diseased condition of the body. But it is our part, as medical missionaries, as workers together with God, to use the means that He has provided. Then we should pray that God will bless these agencies.

457. Practical work is the most useful education in the training of health workers.

Loma Linda Messages, 342.

GREAT care should be exercised in the training of young people for the medical missionary work; for the mind is molded by that which it receives and retains. Too much incomplete work has been done in the education given. The most useful education is that gained by study in connection with practical work.

458. Practical work with health professionals can be beneficial.

Loma Linda Messages, 409.

LET it be more and more deeply impressed upon every student that every one of us should have an intelligent understanding of how to treat the physical system. And there are many who would have greater intelligence in these matters if they would not confine themselves to years of study without a practical experience under the instruction of learned physicians and surgeons.

459. After practical training one should then go out in an apprenticeship with experienced gospel workers.

Loma Linda Messages, 69.

YOUNG men who have a practical knowledge of how to treat the sick are now to be sent out to do gospel medical missionary work, in connection with more experienced gospel workers. If these young men will give themselves to the study of the Word, they will become successful evangelists. The ministers with whom these young men labor are to give them the same opportunity to learn that Elijah gave Elisha. They are to show them how to teach the truth to others. Where it is possible these young men should visit the hospitals, and in some cases they may connect with them for a while, laboring disinterestedly. The purest example of unselfishness is now to be shown by our medical missionary workers. With the knowledge and experience gained by practical work, they are to go out to give treatment to the sick. As they go from house to house, they will find access to many hearts. Many will be reached who otherwise would never have heard the gospel message.

460. Medical missionaries are to be quickly trained in schools outside of the cities.

Loma Linda Messages, 56.

THE Lord calls upon our young people to enter our schools and quickly fit themselves for service. In various places, outside of the cities, schools are to be established, where our youth can receive an education that will prepare them to go forth to do evangelical work and medical missionary work.

461. We are not to train for three to six years before engaging in active work.

Loma Linda Messages, 62–63.

MY BROTHER, I am surprised that you are found asleep on this point. I declare unto you, in the name of the Lord, that the arrangements being made for the training of medical missionaries in Battle Creek are not right. A great work is to be done in a short time, and God forbids that we should encourage so many of our youth to bind themselves up for three, or four, or six years of training, before engaging in active work.

462. Effective medical missionary work can be done by reading and sharing our health literature.

Review and Herald, vol. 4, 369.

THERE is a work to be begun in every city, in every town. What are you going to do to help it forward? You are to obtain all the light and knowledge that you can. There are the health books. Our canvassers can take these books right along with them, and read them. As they go, they will find that there is light in them, which they can present to the families they visit. They will find persons sick, and they can read something in those books that will do these persons good. Many are going to work on this plan. God never sets a man to work, and leaves him without putting any ideas into his mind.

463. We can learn and teach medical missionary work through a home reading circle.

Review and Herald, vol. 4, 439.

MANY who desire to obtain knowledge of medical missionary work have home duties that will sometimes prevent them from meeting with others for study. These may learn much in their own homes in regard to the expressed will of God concerning missionary work, thus increasing their ability to help others. Fathers and mothers, obtain all the help you can from the study of our books and publications. Read the Good Health, for it is full of valuable information. Take time to read to your children from the health books, as well as from the books treating more particularly on religious subjects. Teach them the importance of caring for the body the house they live in. Form a home reading circle, in which every member of the family shall lay aside the busy cares of the day, and unite in study. Fathers, mothers, and brothers, sisters, take up this work heartily, and see if the home church will not be greatly improved.

464. A knowledge of advanced science is power and is needed, but it is not to supersede the knowledge of the gospel in God's final work.

Fundamentals of Christian Education, 186.

A KNOWLEDGE of science of all kinds is power, and it is in the purpose of God that advanced science shall be taught in our schools as a preparation for the work that is to precede the closing scenes of earth's history. The truth is to go to the remotest bounds of the earth, through agents trained for the work. But while the knowledge of science is a power, the knowledge which Jesus in person came to impart to the world was the knowledge of the gospel. The light of truth was to flash its bright rays into the uttermost parts of the earth, and the acceptance or rejection of the message of God involved the eternal destiny of souls.

465. We are to learn all that we can from nature, but we must look to Christ for a knowledge of God's character.

The Youth's Instructor, 107.

IT IS proper to seek to learn all that is possible from nature, but do not fail to look from nature to Christ for the complete representation of the character of the living God.

466. There is a danger in over emphasizing a knowledge of microbes to a neglect of a vital connection with God.

Spalding and Magan, 86.

IF WE had less to say in regard to microbes and more to say in regard to the matchless love and power of God, we would honor God far more. These things are dwelt upon too much, and the things we ought to know, which concern our eternal interest, receive altogether too little attention. Throw a veil over the poor decaying earth, which is corrupted on account of the wickedness of its inhabitants, and point to the heavenly world. There is need of far more teaching in regard to having in this life a vital connection with God through Christ, that we may be fitted to enjoy heaven and dwell forever with our Lord. If we would attain to a pure and elevated ideal of character, we must lift up Jesus, the perfect example; the exalting of science will never accomplish the work.

467. The Lord will have for those who are perfecting Christian characters a place to work in true missionary lines.

Loma Linda Messages, 60.

OUR churches who have a deep interest in the children and youth, and in the work of training workers to carry forward the work essential for this time, need not blunder; for God will open ways before all who are perfecting Christian characters. He will have places ready for them in which to begin to do true missionary work. It was to prepare workers for this work, that our schools and sanitariums were established.

468. Every health institution is to train medical missionaries.

Testimonies, vol. 7, 100.

CAUTIONS have been given me in reference to the work of training nurses and medical missionary evangelists. We are not to centralize this work in any one place. In every sanitarium established, young men and young women should be trained to be medical missionaries. The Lord will open the way before them as they go forth to work for Him.

469. Every church is to instruct its members in medical missionary work.

Testimonies, vol. 7, 112–113.

IN EVERY place where there is a church, instruction should be given in regard to the preparation of simple, healthful foods for the use of those who wish to live in accordance with the principles of health reform. And the church members should impart to the people of their neighborhood the light they receive on this subject.

470. Those who do not believe the Word of God cannot train acceptable medical missionaries.

Loma Linda Messages, 545.

I AM charged to present these Scriptures to our people, that they may understand that those who do not believe the Word of God cannot possibly present to those who desire to become acceptable medical missionaries, the way by which they will become most successful. Christ was the greatest Physician the world has ever known; His heart was ever touched with human woe. He has a work for those to do who will not place their dependence upon worldly powers.

471. We should fear to place ourselves under the influence of worldly teachers.

Loma Linda Messages, 543.

I WAS shown that now in a special sense we as a people are to be guided by divine instruction. Those fitting themselves for medical missionary work should fear to place themselves under the direction of worldly doctors, to imbibe their sentiments and peculiar prejudices, and to learn to express their ideas and views. They are not to depend for their influence upon worldly teachers. They should be "looking unto Jesus, the author and finisher of our faith."

472. Intelligent medical missionary work will serve as entering-wedge credentials for our religious principles.

Healthful Living, 273.

THE field for medical missionary work is open before us. We are now beginning to comprehend the light given years ago that health reform principles would form an entering wedge to the introduction of religious principles. To voice the words of John, "Behold the Lamb of God that taketh away the sin of the world." Would that all our workers might be enlightened, so that they could work intelligently as medical missionaries, for such knowledge would serve as credentials to them in finding access to homes and families wherein to sow the seeds of truth.

473. Much good can be done by those with less training who are working under competent physicians.

Special Testimonies, Series B, 214.

MUCH good can be done by those who do not hold diplomas as fully accredited physicians. Some are to be prepared to work as competent physicians. Many, working under the direction of such ones, can do acceptable work without spending so long a time in studying as it has been thought necessary to spend in the past.

474. Our methods of training in the use of God's remedies were to be recognized as preferable to methods demanding poisonous drugs.

Loma Linda Messages, 365.

IN THE work of the school maintain simplicity. No argument is so powerful as is success founded upon simplicity. And you may attain success in the education of students as medical missionaries without a medical school that can qualify physicians to compete with the physicians of the world.

Let the students be given a practical education. And the less dependent you are upon worldly methods of education, the better it will be for the students. Special instruction should be given in the art of treating the sick without the use of poisonous drugs, and in harmony with the light that God has given. Students should come forth from the school without having sacrificed the principles of health reform.

The education that meets the world's standard is to be less and less valued by those who are seeking for efficiency in carrying the medical missionary work in connection with the work of the third angel's message. They are to be educated from the standpoint of conscience; and as they conscientiously and faithfully follow right methods in their treatment of the sick, these methods will come to be recognized as preferable to the method of nursing to which many have been accustomed, which demands the use of poisonous drugs.

475. We are to depend upon the power of God to impress minds, rather than upon the world's acknowledgement.

Loma Linda Messages, 409.

YOU may say, the world will not acknowledge us. What if the world will not acknowledge you? It is the power of God that makes the impress on the human mind.

476. The same Jesus who daily taught His disciples will teach wisdom to His servants in this age.

Loma Linda Messages, 414.

TEACH the students to look for wisdom to the One who gave His life for the salvation of the world. Now is your time to work. That same Jesus who walked with His disciples on earth, and who taught them from day to day, will teach His servants in this age.

477. Those under the instruction of the Great Medical Missionary will receive knowledge that the world cannot supply.

Loma Linda Messages, 66.

AND the needed knowledge will be given to all who come to Christ, receiving and practicing His teachings, making His words a part of their lives. Those who place themselves under the instruction of the great Medical Missionary, to be workers together with Him, will have a knowledge that

The Final Work

the world, with all its traditional lore, cannot supply.

478. Workers must depend upon God for wisdom and power, and not upon man.

Loma Linda Messages, 58.

LET the workers remember always that they are dependent on God. Let them not trust in human wisdom, but in the wisdom of the One who declares, "All power is given unto me in heaven and in earth. . . . Lo, I am with you alway, even unto the end of the world." Let them go forth two and two, depending upon God, not on man, for wisdom and success. Let them search the Scriptures, and then present the truths of God's Word to others. Let them be guided by the principles that Christ has laid down.

479. Every health-restoring work must be tested by the Holy Scriptures.

Maranatha, 156.

THE last great delusion is soon to open before us. Antichrist is to perform his marvelous works in our sight. So closely will the counterfeit resemble the true that it will be impossible to distinguish between them except by the Holy Scriptures. By their testimony every statement and every miracle must be tested.

480. True experience will be in perfect harmony with natural and divine law.

Testimonies, vol. 3, 72–73.

EVE ate and imagined that she felt the sensations of a new and more exalted life. She bore the fruit to her husband, and that which had an overpowering influence upon him was her experience. The serpent had said that she should not die, and she felt no ill effects from the fruit, nothing which could be interpreted to mean death, but, just as the serpent had said, a pleasurable sensation which she imagined was as the angels felt. Her experience stood arrayed against the positive command of Jehovah, and Adam permitted himself to be seduced by the experience of his wife.

A true experience will be in perfect harmony with natural and divine law. False experience will array itself against science and the principles of Jehovah.

481. When there is not a "Thus saith the Lord" our health-care methods must be based on actual experiment and thorough investigation, rather than upon "personal experience."

The Health Reformer, 78–79.

EXPERIENCE is said to be the best teacher. Genuine experience is indeed valuable. . . . But true experience is in harmony with natural law and science. . . .

Genuine experience is a variety of experiments entered into carefully, with the mind freed from prejudice and uncontrolled by previously established opinions and habits; marking the results with careful solicitude, anxious to learn, improve, and reform, on every or any habit, if that habit is not in harmony with physical and moral law. With some, the idea of others gainsaying that which they have learned by experience seems to them to be folly, and even cruelty itself. But there are more

errors received, and firmly retained, under the false idea of experience, than from any other cause. For this reason, that which is generally termed experience is no experience at all, because there has never been a fair trial by actual experiment and thorough investigation, with a knowledge of the principle involved in the action. . . .

Genuine experience is in harmony with the unchangeable principles of nature. Superstition, caused by diseased imagination, is frequently in conflict with science and principle. And yet the unanswerable argument is urged, "I must be correct, for this is my experience." There are many invalids today who will ever remain so, because they cannot be convinced that their experience is not reliable.

482. Medical missionary work must be carried forward with a greater earnestness than ever before.

Loma Linda Messages, 63.

THERE are souls in many places who have not yet heard the message. Henceforth medical missionary work is to be carried forward with an earnestness with which it has never yet been done.

483. Today the Lord is qualifying those who are willing to follow Him for medical missionary work.

Spalding and Magan, 427.

TODAY the Lord is qualifying His servants to take up medical missionary work. He calls for men and women who are peaceable in spirit, who learn of Jesus, and are willing to follow His instruction, who day by day wait upon the Lord to know His will, prepared to go where He bids them go, and to take up the work which He requires.

484. God calls for one thousand medical missionary workers where now there is one.

Battle Creek Letters, 114.

A WORLD is perishing in sin, and God calls for workers. He wants one thousand at work in the highways and in the hedges, where now there is but one. We have no time to listen to idle tales and false science. The faith of many will be revived when they will humble their hearts before God, and go forth to fulfill the commission of Christ, "Go ye into all the world, and preach the gospel to every creature."

485. A fitness for the work is imparted as we answer, "Here am I; send me."

Bible Echo, September 18, 1899.

GOD has His workmen in every age. The call of the hour is answered by the human agencies. Thus it will be when the divine voice cries, "Whom shall I send? and who will go for us?" The response will come, "Here am I, send me." The Lord imparts a fitness for the work to every man and woman who will cooperate with divine power. A great work is to be done in our world, and human agencies will surely respond to the demand. And all the requisite talent, courage, perseverance, faith, and tact will come as they put the armor on. The world must hear the warning. When the call comes, "Whom shall I send, and who will go for us?" send back the answer clear and distinct, "Here am I; send me."

Health Reform / Deform

486. Two purposes of health reform are to relieve suffering and to purify the church.

Testimonies, vol. 9, 112–113.

THE work of health reform is the Lord's means for lessening suffering in our world and for purifying His church.

487. The acceptance or rejection of the principles of health reform has eternal consequences for they are an essential part of present truth.

Elder J. H. Waggoner, *Review and Herald*, August 7, 1866. (*The Story of Our Health Message*, 79–80)

WE DO not profess to be pioneers in the general principles of the health reform. The facts on which this movement is based have been elaborated, in a great measure, by reformers, physicians, and writers on physiology and hygiene, and so may be found scattered through the land. But we do claim that by the method of God's choice it has been more clearly and powerfully unfolded, and is thereby producing an effect which we could not have looked for from any other means.

As mere physiological and hygienic truths, they might be studied by some at their leisure, and by others laid aside as of little consequence; but when placed on a level with the great truths of the third angel's message by the sanction and authority of God's Spirit, and so declared to be the means whereby a weak people may be made strong to overcome, and our diseased bodies cleansed and fitted for translation, then it comes to us as an essential part of present truth, to be received with the blessing of God, or rejected at our peril.

488. Health reform reveals the sinfulness of violating natural law.

Counsels on Health, 21.

MEN and women cannot violate natural law by indulging depraved appetites and lustful passions, without violating the law of God. Therefore He has permitted the light of health reform to shine upon us, that we may realize the sinfulness of breaking the laws which He has established in our being.

489. A perfect life without sin includes obedience to the natural laws of the body.

Counsels on Health, 20.

When men take any course which needlessly expends their vitality or beclouds their intellect, they sin against God; they do not glorify Him in their body and spirit, which are His. Yet despite the insult which man has offered Him, God's love is still extended to the race; and He permits light to shine, enabling man to see that in order to live a perfect life he must obey the natural laws which govern his being. How important, then, that man should walk in this light, exercising all his powers, both of body and mind, to the glory of God!

490. Health reform is an essential part of the message to prepare for Christ's coming.

Counsels on Health, 20–21.

THE health reform is one branch of the great work which is to fit a people for the coming of the Lord. It is as closely connected with the third angel's message as the hand is with the body.

491. The practice and teaching of health reform will lead others to investigate spiritual truths.

Evangelism, 514.

I HAVE been informed by my guide that not only should those who believe the truth practice health reform but they should also teach it diligently to others; for it will be an agency through which the truth can be presented to the attention of unbelievers. They will reason that if we have such sound ideas in regard to health and temperance, there must be something in our religious belief that is worth investigation. If we backslide in health reform we shall lose much of our influence with the outside world.

492. All can utilize health reform to do the Lord's work.

Testimonies, vol. 9, 112–113.

THE work of health reform is the Lord's means for lessening suffering in our world and for purifying His church. Teach the people that they can act as God's helping hand by cooperating with the Master Worker in restoring physical and spiritual health. This work bears the signature of heaven and will open doors for the entrance of other precious truths. There is room for all to labor who will take hold of this work intelligently.

493. We are neither to reject health reform nor are we to be too rigid in our personal ideas of how to apply it.

Counsels on Diet and Foods, 196.

TWO classes have been presented before me: first, those who are not living up to the light which God has given them; secondly, those who are too rigid in carrying out their one-sided ideas of reform, and enforcing them on others. When they take a position, they stand to it stubbornly, and carry nearly everything over the mark.

494. Extreme views of health reform have irreversible spiritual consequences.

Counsels on Health, 153–154.

WHEN those who advocate hygienic reform carry the matter to extremes, people are not to blame if they become disgusted. Too often our religious faith is thus brought into disrepute, and in many cases those who witness such exhibitions of inconsistency can never afterward be brought to think that there is anything good in the reform. These extremists do more harm in a few months than they can undo in a lifetime. They are engaged in a work which Satan loves to see go on.

495. Satan brings extremists in among us to discredit us as a body.

Medical Ministry, 269.

IT IS the desire and plan of Satan to bring in among us those who will go to great extremes—people of narrow minds, who are critical and sharp, and very tenacious in holding their own conceptions of what the truth means. They will be exacting, and will seek to enforce rigorous duties, and go to great length in matters of minor importance, while they neglect the weightier matters of the law—judgment and mercy and the love of God. Through the work of a few of this class of persons, the whole body of Sabbathkeepers will be designated as bigoted, pharisaical, and fanatical. The work of the truth, because of these workers, will be thought to be unworthy of notice.

496. Extremes in health reform are health deform.

Counsels on Diet and Foods, 202.

I HAVE something to say in reference to extreme views of health reform. Health reform becomes health deform, a health destroyer, when it is carried to extremes.

497. Cooking all food like vegetables prepared only with water is health deform.

Counsels on Diet and Foods, 212.

I HAVE been where these radical ideas have been carried out. Vegetables prepared with only water, and everything else in like manner. This kind of cookery is health deform, and there are some minds so constituted that they will accept anything that bears the features of rigorous diet or reform of any kind.

498. A low quality and quantity of food is health deform.

Testimonies, vol. 6, 374.

IT IS contrary to health reform, after cutting off the great variety of unwholesome dishes, to go to the opposite extreme, reducing the quantity and quality of the food to a low standard. Instead of health reform this is health deform.

499. Overeating of even health foods is health deform.

Manuscript Releases, vol. 8, 175.

WITH many, health reform means nothing more than to live without the use of flesh meat. The so-called health reform of many might be better termed health deform. There is too much eating merely to gratify the appetite. Because the foods are called health foods and are appetizing, some think it proper to eat more than they should. God desires us to restrain our appetites. We should partake of simple food, and eat no more than the stomach can readily take care of.

500. We are not to present to God's people diet teachings that are strained to the farthest point of extension.

Counsels on Diet and Foods, 205.

GOD calls upon those for whom Christ died to take proper care of themselves, and set a right example to others. My brother, you are not to make a test for the people of God, upon the question of diet; for they will lose confidence in teachings that are strained to the farthest point of extension. The Lord desires His people to be sound on every point in health reform, but we must not go to extremes.

501. Reforms strained to the highest tension will lead some to adopt unhealthful practices.

Counsels on Diet and Foods, 206.

THE reforms that are strained to the highest tension might accommodate a certain class, who can obtain all they need to take the place of the things discarded; but this class forms a very small minority of the people to whom these tests seem unnecessary. There are those who try to abstain from what is declared to be harmful. They fail to supply the system with proper nourishment, and as a consequence become weak and unable to work.

502. Extremists are in danger of preparing unappetizing food resulting in poor nutrition.

Testimonies, vol. 9, 161–162.

SOME of our people, while conscientiously abstaining from eating improper foods, neglect to supply themselves with the elements necessary for the sustenance of the body. Those who take an extreme view of health reform are in danger of preparing tasteless dishes, making them so insipid that they are not satisfying. Food should be prepared in such a way that it will be appetizing as well as nourishing. It should not be robbed of that which the system needs. I use some salt, and always have, because salt, instead of being deleterious, is actually essential for the blood. Vegetables should be made palatable with a little milk or cream, or something equivalent.

503. A continual sameness in diet and poorly prepared food which is unappetizing is not health reform.

Testimonies, vol. 2, 63.

I AM acquainted with families who have changed from a meat diet to one that is impoverished. Their food is so poorly prepared that the stomach loathes it; and such have told me that the health reform did not agree with them, that they were decreasing in physical strength. Here is one reason why some have not been successful in their efforts to simplify their food. They have a poverty-stricken diet. Food is prepared without painstaking, and there is a continual sameness. There should not be many kinds at any one meal, but all meals should not be composed of the same kinds of food without variation. Food should be prepared with simplicity, yet with a nicety which will invite the appetite.

504. We should avoid personal views that result in leaving out of the diet nourishment which the system needs.

Counsels on Diet and Foods, 203.

AT ONE time Doctor _____ tried to teach our family to cook according to health reform, as he viewed it, without salt or anything else to season the food. Well, I determined to try it, but I became so reduced in strength that I had to make a change; and a different policy was entered upon with great success. I tell you this because I know that you are in positive danger. Food should be prepared in such a way that it will be nourishing. It should not be robbed of that which the system needs.

505. Some have followed extremes in diet resulting in the weakening of the temple of God.

Testimonies, vol. 1, 205.

SOME have gone to extremes in regard to diet. They have taken a rigid course, and lived so very plain that their health has suffered, disease has strengthened in the system, and the temple of God has been weakened.

506. The extremes of unwise minds disgusts rather than converts others to health reform.

Counsels on Diet and Foods, 212.

THE great backsliding upon health reform is because unwise minds have handled it and carried it to such extremes that it has disgusted in place of converting people to it.

507. Avoid fanatical extremes while setting an example in the adoption of health reform.

Counsels on Diet and Foods, 366.

DO NOT go to extremes in regard to the health reform. Some of our people are very careless in regard to health reform. But because some are far behind, you must not, in order to be an example to them, be an extremist. You must not deprive yourself of that class of food which makes good blood. Your devotion to true principles is leading you to submit yourself to a diet which is giving you an experience that will not recommend health reform.

508. Innovations to the principles of health reform will lead conscientious souls to extreme practices injurious to the cause of health reform.

Counsels on Diet and Foods, 352.

THERE is danger that in presenting the principles of health reform some will be in favor of bringing in changes that would be for the worse instead of for the better. Health reform must not be urged in a radical manner. We must be careful to make no innovations, because under the influence of extreme teaching there are conscientious souls who will surely go to extremes. Their physical appearance will injure the cause of health reform; for few know how to properly supply the place of that which they discard.

509. The best qualified advocates will be unable to fully undo the prejudice created by extremists.

Testimonies, vol. 2, 386–387.

IT IS impossible for the best qualified advocates of health reform to fully relieve the minds of the public from the prejudice received through the wrong course of these extremists and to place the great subject of health reform upon a right basis in the community where these men have figured. The door is also closed in a great measure, so that unbelievers cannot be reached by the present truth upon the Sabbath and the soon coming of our Saviour. The most precious truths are cast aside by the people as unworthy of a hearing. These men are referred to as representatives of health reformers and Sabbathkeepers in general. A great responsibility rests upon those who have thus proved a stumbling block to unbelievers.

510. Our own opinions produce human tests which work against God's health reform message.

Counsels on Diet and Foods, 209–210.

THE church and the world need all the influence, all the talents God has given us. All we have should be appropriated to His use. In presenting the gospel, keep out all your own opinions. We have a worldwide message, and the Lord wants His servants to guard sacredly the trust He has given them. To every man God has given his work. Then let no false message be borne. Let there be no straining into inconsistent problems the grand light of health reform. The inconsistencies of one rest upon the whole body of believers; therefore when one goes to extremes, great harm is done to the cause of God.

The carrying of things to extremes is a matter to be dreaded. It always results in my being compelled to speak to prevent matters from being misunderstood, so that the world will not have cause to think that Seventh-day Adventists are a body of extremists. When we seek to pull people out of the fire on the one hand, the very words which then have to be spoken to correct evils are used to justify indulgence on the other hand. May the Lord keep us from human tests and extremes.

511. Let us not labor to raise others to personal false standards.

Testimonies, vol. 2, 374–375.

AND while we would caution you not to overeat, even of the best quality of food, we would also caution those that are extremists not to raise a false standard and then endeavor to bring everybody to it.

512. God has other ways for us to reveal our humility than by man-made crosses in health reform.

Testimonies, vol. 1, 205–206.

I SAW that God does not require anyone to take a course of such rigid economy as to weaken or injure the temple of God. There are duties and requirements in His word to humble the church and cause them to afflict their souls, and there is no need of making crosses and manufacturing duties to distress the body in order to cause humility. All this is outside of the word of God.

513. The starvation plan will not make us spiritually

minded nor glorify God.

Our High Calling, 265.

IT IS our duty to train and discipline the body in order that we shall render to the Master the highest possible service. Inclination must not control us. We are not to pamper the appetite and indulge in the use of that which is not for our good, simply because it gratifies the palate; neither are we to seek to live by the starvation plan, with the idea that we shall become spiritually-minded, and that God shall be glorified. We must use the intelligence that God has given in order that we may be perfect in body, soul, and spirit, that we may have a symmetrical character, a well-balanced mind, and do perfect work for the Master.

514. Our health reform message must be God's message.

Counsels on Diet and Foods, 210.

I WAS instructed to say to those in the _____ Conference who had been so strenuous upon the subject of health reform, urging their ideas and views upon others, that God had not given them their message.

515. We must not laden men with burdens grievous to be borne.

LUKE 11:46.

WOE unto you . . . for ye lade men with burdens grievous to be borne.

516. The church is crippled when things that God has not required are promoted.

Counsels on Diet and Foods, 206.

HEALTH reform is brought to disrepute. The work we have tried to build up solidly is confused with strange things that God has not required. The energies of the church are crippled.

517. If we err from the middle path it should be on the side of the people.

Counsels on Diet and Foods, 211.

IF YOU err, let it not be in getting as far from the people as possible, for then you cut the thread of your influence and can do them no good. Better err on the side of the people than altogether away from them, for there is hope in that case that you can carry the people with you, but there is no need of error on either side.

You need not go into the water, or into the fire, but take the middle path, avoiding all extremes. Do not let it appear that you are one-sided, ill-balanced managers. Do not have a meager, poor diet. Do not let anyone influence you to have the diet poverty-stricken. Have your food prepared in a healthful, tasteful manner; have your food prepared with a nicety that will correctly represent health reform.

518. It is best to come short of the mark than to go beyond it.

Testimonies, vol. 3, 21.

IN REFORMS we would better come one step short of the mark than to go one step beyond it. And if there is error at all, let it be on the side next to the people.

519. Advances in health reform are to progress only as the earlier phases are done well.

Testimonies, vol. 7, 135.

IN TEACHING health reform, as in all other gospel work, we are to meet the people where they are. Until we can teach them how to prepare health reform foods that are palatable, nourishing, and yet inexpensive, we are not at liberty to present the most advanced propositions regarding health reform diet. Let the diet reform be progressive.

520. Presenting first the strongest positions will discourage some from making changes.

Testimonies, vol. 3, 21.

IF WE come to persons who have not been enlightened in regard to health reform, and present our strongest positions at first, there is danger of their becoming discouraged as they see how much they have to give up, so that they will make no effort to reform. We must lead the people along patiently and gradually, remembering the hole of the pit whence we were digged.

521. The ill may initially require a strict diet but this should be liberalized as health improves.

Counsels on Diet and Foods, 207.

SOME may come to the sanitarium in a condition demanding stern denial of appetite and the simplest fare, but as their health improves, they should be liberally supplied with nourishing food.

522. Our present diet should strengthen us for the time of trouble when a more restrictive diet will be required.

Counsels on Diet and Foods, 202.

THEY (God's people) should seek rest of body and mind from wearing labor when they can, and should eat of nourishing, strengthening food to build up their strength; for they will be obliged to exercise all the strength they have. I saw that it does not glorify God in the least for any of His people to make a time of trouble for themselves. . . .

The time of trouble is just before us; and then stern necessity will require the people of God to deny self, and to eat merely enough to sustain life; but God will prepare us for that time.

523. Our health habits should be as much like others as possible without sacrificing principle.

The Ministry of Healing, 324.

HYGIENISTS should not try to see how different they can be from others, but should come as near to them as possible without the sacrifice of principle.

Testimonies, vol. 1, 456.

NO occasion should be given to unbelievers to reproach our faith. We are considered odd and singular, and should not take a course to lead unbelievers to think us more so than our faith requires us to be.

524. While avoiding fanaticism we must still be firm and decided for right.

The Ministry of Healing, 324.

HYGIENIC reform is based upon principles that are broad and far-reaching, and we should not belittle it by narrow views and practices. But no one should permit opposition or ridicule, or a desire to please or influence others, to turn him from true principles, or cause him lightly to regard them. Those who are governed by principle will be firm and decided in standing for the right; yet in all their associations they will manifest a generous, Christlike spirit and true moderation.

525. We must leave room for the Holy Spirit to work.

Fundamentals of Christian Education, 363.

LET educators give the Holy Spirit room to do its work upon human hearts.

526. We must leave room for Christ to minister to those who are following Him.

Selected Messages, book 1, 178.

THE soul that accepts Jesus places himself under the care of the Great Physician, and let men be careful how they come between the patient and the Physician who discerns all the needs of the soul. . . . But men are so officious, they want to do so much, that they overdo the matter, leaving Christ no room to work.

527. Because of differences in food tolerances each one must discover how best to have a healthful diet.

Counsels on Diet and Foods, 494.

THERE is a wide difference in constitutions and temperaments, and the demands of the system differ greatly in different persons. What would be food for one, might be poison for another; so precise rules cannot be laid down to fit every case. I cannot eat beans, for they are poison to me; but for me to say that for this reason no one must eat them would be simply ridiculous. I cannot eat a spoonful of milk gravy, or milk toast, without suffering in consequence; but other members of my family can eat these things, and realize no such effect; therefore I take that which suits my stomach best, and they do the same. We have no words, no contention; all moves along harmoniously in my large family, for I do not attempt to dictate what they shall or shall not eat.

528. Providing a variety of simple, wholesome, palatable food will permit each to choose what is individually best without controversy.

Counsels on Diet and Foods, 491.

I EAT the most simple food, prepared in the most simple way. For months my principal diet has been vermicelli and canned tomatoes, cooked together. This I eat with zwieback. Then I have also stewed fruit of some kind and sometimes lemon pie. Dried corn, cooked with milk or a little cream, is another dish that I sometimes use.

But the other members of my family do not eat the same things that I do. I do not hold myself up as a criterion for them. I leave each one to follow his own ideas as to what is best for him. I bind no one else's conscience by my own. One person cannot be a criterion for another in the matter of eating. It is impossible to make one rule for all to follow. . . . Butter is never placed on my table, but if the members of my family choose to use a little butter away from the table, they are at liberty to do so. Our table is set twice a day, but if there are those who desire something to eat in the evening, there is no rule that forbids them from getting it. No one complains or goes from our table dissatisfied. A variety of food that is simple, wholesome, and palatable, is always provided.

529. We need to avoid one-idea fanaticism.

Selected Messages, book 2, 319.

THESE one-idea men can see nothing except to press the one thing that presents itself to their minds. . . .

Now we read in the Bible of a good conscience; and there are not only good but bad consciences. There is a conscientiousness that will carry everything to extremes, and make Christian duties as burdensome as the Jews made the observance of the Sabbath. . . . One fanatic, with his strong spirit and radical ideas, who will oppress the conscience of those who want to be right, will do great harm. The church needs to be purified from all such influences.

530. We can maintain confidence in health reform through the avoidance of extremes if we follow God rather than man.

Counsels on Diet and Foods, 211.

BROTHER and Sister _____ carried the matter of indulgence in eating to extreme, and the institute became demoralized. Now the enemy would push you into the opposite extreme if he could, to have a poverty-stricken diet. Be careful to keep level heads and sensible ideas. Seek wisdom from heaven and move understandingly. If you take extremely radical positions, you will be obliged to back down, and then however conscientious you may have been you have lost confidence in your own sound judgment, and our brethren and unbelievers will lose confidence in you. Be sure to go no faster than you have positive light from God. Take no man's ideas, but move intelligently in the fear of the Lord.

531. God will intervene to counteract the results of the strenuous ideas that He has not required.

Testimonies, vol. 9, 162.

THE work that we have tried to build up solidly is confused with strange things that God has not required, and the energies of the church are crippled. But God will interfere to prevent the results of these too strenuous ideas.

532. God promises that His health reform program will be presented with great success.

Medical Ministry, 271.

THE Lord has presented before me that many, many will be rescued from physical, mental, and moral degeneracy through the practical influence of health reform. Health talks will be given, publications will be multiplied. The principles of health reform will be received with favor; and many will be enlightened. The influences that are associated with health reform will commend it to the judgment of all who want light; and they will advance step by step to receive the special truths for this time.

533. Obedience to God led to no "feebleness" in Israel during the forty years in the wilderness.

Desire of Ages, 824.

CHRIST had been the guide and teacher of ancient Israel, and He taught them that health is the reward of obedience to the laws of God. The Great Physician who healed the sick in Palestine had spoken to His people from the pillar of cloud, telling them what they must do, and what God would do for them. "If thou wilt diligently hearken to the voice of the Lord thy God," He said, "and wilt do that which is right in His sight, and wilt give ear to His commandments, and keep all His statutes, I will put none of these diseases upon thee, which I have brought upon the Egyptians: for I am the Lord that healeth thee." Ex. 15:26. Christ gave to Israel definite instruction in regard to their habits of life, and He assured them, "The Lord will take away from thee all sickness." Deut. 7:15. When they fulfilled the conditions, the promise was verified to them. "There was not one feeble person among their tribes." Ps. 105:37.

534. There are invalids due to no fault of their own.

Manuscript Releases, vol. 9, 281.

THERE are invalids in our world born with feeble constitutions. They suffer from no fault of their own. Let these study patient endurance. In so doing they can glorify God.

535. Though the Christian may suffer a lingering illness in this life, through divine grace, he can cheerfully bear it.

Review and Herald, April 28, 1859.

THE Christian is subject to sickness, disappointment, poverty, reproach and distress. Yet amid all this he loves God, and loves to do his will, and prizes nothing so highly as his approbation. In the conflicts, trials, and changing scenes of this life, he knows that there is One who understands it all; One who will bend his ear low to the cries of the sorrowful and distressed; One who can sympathize with every sorrow and soothe the keenest anguish of every heart. He has invited the sorrowing ones to come to him and find rest. Amid all his affliction the Christian has strong consolation, and if he suffers a lingering, distressing sickness, before he closes his eyes in death, he can with cheerfulness bear it all, for he holds communion with his Redeemer. You often see his countenance radiant with joy, while he contemplates the future with heavenly satisfaction—only a short rest in the grave, and the Life-giver will break the fetters of the tomb, release the captive and bring him from his dusty bed immortal, never more to know pain, sorrow or death. Let this hope of the Christian be our hope, and we will ask no more.

536. The Christian will be fully free from sickness only in the future life.

Manuscript Releases, vol. 3, 107.

THIS earth is the place of preparation for heaven. The time spent here is the Christian's winter. Here the chilly winds of affliction blow upon us, and the waves of trouble roll against us. But in the near future, when Christ comes, sorrow and sighing will be forever ended. Then will be the Christian's summer. All trials will be over, and there will be no more sickness or death. "God shall wipe away all tears from their eyes, and there shall be no more death, neither shall there be any more pain; for the former things have passed away."